Beauty

Vitality

Longevity

$SIZE\ \underline{2}\ FOR\ LIFE$

The amazingly simple diet and fitness plan to transform your shape forever!

by

Ashley Marriott and Marc L. Paulsen, M.D.

Size 2 for Life: The amazingly simple diet and fitness plan to transform your shape forever!

By: Ashley Marriott and Marc L. Paulsen, M.D.

www.stancepublications.com

Fitness models: Ashley Marriott, Justine Javelle, Ashley Spence and Monique Burgee

Photography by Marc Paulsen and Anacia Weiskittel

Publisher: Stance Publications
Newport Beach, California

ISBN 978-0-9821047-4-3

Note to Readers

Table of Contents

Foreword

by

Marc L. Paulsen, M.D.

You didn't start life as a size 8, 12, 16 or more. So how did you get here? Well, the simple fact is you ate, and you ate and year after year you ate. Brilliant, right? Now you're saying "tell me something that I don't already know before I chuck this book and go back to the nachos!" Well sorry, what I'm actually going to tell you is something you also already know: You need to eat less AND you need to exercise (ugh!) if you really want to spend your life as a size 2. But, you might logically state, "I've already tried all the 'supercharged' diets, the 'spot reduction' diets, the celebrity diets, all without success. What does this plan have to offer that they didn't?" Well, the facts are that brief interval exercise programs are insufficient to result in any real and sustained weight loss while spot reduction programs have no legitimate basis.

In *Size 2 for Life,* what we give you is a simple and realistic diet and exercise program that almost anyone can follow – with the emphasis on simple. But, from the outset, although we can make things as easy as possible, you need to understand that sustained weight loss requires a lifestyle change that includes healthy eating and regular exercise. If you're not willing to make this (almost) daily concession, you might as well go back to the nachos. On the other hand, we truly believe that if you make the minor lifestyle adjustments and follow our program, you can realistically spend your life as a frame adjusted size 2 (more on that later).

Some people have asked us why we chose such a politically incorrect title. They even go so far as to warn us about the potential backlash it could create. Others ask, quite correctly, whether or not we agree that excessive thinness is unhealthy. To the later I respond that I absolutely agree. But the fact is that a frame adjusted size 2 is *not* excessive thinness. Although the lower limit of healthy body fat percentage in women is a hotly debated subject, many researchers have found that slim, trim, athletic and healthy women commonly maintain total body fat percentages of 17 – 22% or less without suffering any ill effects.[1] In fact, there is ample evidence to show that there are substantial benefits to maintaining a healthy range of body fat including reduced risk for cancer, heart disease, diabetes and stroke. It's a lean, trim and athletic physique that not only garners attention but also leads to a longer and higher quality life. But what is also blatantly true is that the current "plus size acceptance mentality" is dangerous and, as a medical professional, I feel the personal obligation to accept the challenge of political incorrectness and promote the cause of health.

---

[1] William D. McArdle, Frank J. Katch, Victor L. Katch, *Exercise Physiology, Energy, Nutrition & Human Performance*, Sixth Edition, 2007 Chapter 28: "Body Composition Assessment."

Some plus size women claim that they're happy with their weight but it's my belief that this is mostly a defensive ruse. Most women that I've had as patients don't want to be overweight or obese. But what's happened in the majority of these cases is that the varied responsibilities and unanticipated complexities of life have progressively led them into a lifestyle of unhealthy living and lack of exercise. Furthermore, women are constantly barraged with highly promoted, easy fix diet plans, whose abbreviated programs serve only the purpose of selling more books.

We hope that women will approach our book with an open mind and a true sense of determination. We are completely confident that if they follow the program outlined in the book that they will truly achieve a (frame adjusted) size 2 along with all of its rewards.

A brief note on formatting

The book is largely a cooperative work by Ashley Marriott and Marc Paulsen, M.D. In areas where a particular author wishes to emphasize her/his personal perspective the segment will appear *in italics*. Also, scattered throughout the book we have the good fortune of some wonderful women who have been willing to share their journey to size 2 with all of us. Their boxed quotes are greatly appreciated.

> *"I am and have always been a size 2… As a spa and wellness travel writer and editor, I walk-the-talk and live a lifestyle which has allowed me to keep super slim and healthy. The bonus is that I have unlimited energy, plus people always think I'm younger than I am." - Anne Dimon, Founder/Editor, www.traveltowellness.com*

Introduction

As you can imagine, *Size 2 for Life* is a title that can elicit strong reactions such as: anger (throwing this book at the first size 2 woman you see), excitement (opening the book frantically looking for the page with the magic supplement information) or curiosity ("Why would I want to be a size 2?" "Is this a joke?" "Isn't that unrealistic or even unhealthy?").

For us the title is significant in its value as a triple-entendre, offering not only the ability to achieve the best shape you can, but to enjoy your new found health throughout a wonderfully improved and also extended lifetime. I hope that even if you've had any or all of the reactions listed above you'll continue to read further because the information in this book will empower you, educate you and inspire you to realize your true physical as well as emotional potential knowing that a healthy body feeds and sustains a healthy mind.

Many women are aware that the notion of size has changed over the last half century. This applies to both portion sizes and clothing sizes. *Size 2 for Life* is about attaining and maintaining the best physical version of you possible. To do this, which I know you can, you need information, inspiration, and targeted perspiration.

Helping women (sorry guys, you're on your own) reach their fitness goals has been my honor and passion for the last 15 years. It's been inspiring to help hundreds of woman transform themselves through exercise and healthy eating, but it's important to note that many of them began the process with a list of common limiting, destructive and false beliefs including the following:

- I'll never be thin
- My whole family is big
- I don't like to exercise
- I just had a baby, I'll never be a size 2
- I feel selfish if I leave to workout
- My kids won't eat it if I cook "healthy"
- I'm just at my *weight set point*
- If I'm thin people will think I'm vain
- It doesn't matter what I eat or if I exercise I'm large boned

We're a nation addicted to excuses. The fact is obesity rates are at an epidemic; soon to overtake tobacco use as the #1 cause of preventable death. Women are being lied to by clothing companies who are using "vanity sizes" to keep consumers in denial. Food companies are filling us with processed non-foods and pharmaceutical companies are making fortunes selling us pills to manage the illnesses we're getting from our poor diets and lack of exercise. We may not have control over the mass marketing of obesity inducing crap, but we do have control over what we choose to eat and whether or not we choose to exercise.

Now let's take a look at some popular myths before we get started on our journey to size 2.

Size 2 Myths

Myth #1: A Size 2 is a Size 2.

Shopping for clothes these days can feel like a game, "What size will I fit today?" A size 8 at the GAP could be a size 6 at Anne Taylor, and YIPIEE, you're a size 4 at Target. If you find yourself bewildered and can't figure out what size you really are, you're not alone. How can we know what size we are when there's no Standardized Size in the US?

In the 1940's US standard clothing sizes were actually set, but as Americans we've "out grown" those standard sizes. The clothing companies have kept us happy with the number on the tag over the past seventy years by the use of "vanity sizing." Yes, "vanity sizing" has literally manipulated, for example, a size 12 into a size 6.

Through the use of "vanity sizing" we've been able to "super size" our meals and expand our waistlines yet somehow keep wearing the same size pants. Savvy clothing manufacturers understand that women prefer buying smaller sizes and don't want to move into "plus sizes." We've also seen the creation of a size 0 and even a size 00! This is due to the fact that thin women, who in the past may have worn size 2, 4 or even 6, have been "downsized" to the size 0. What's next the -1?

Travel to other parts of the world where this feel good size manipulation has not infiltrated clothing tags and you'll realize we are, in large part, a nation in denial of our true sizes. Think about the icon Marilyn Monroe, often referred to as a curvy size 12, but her measurements 35-22-35 are much closer to today's size 2. The fact is we're experiencing an obesity crisis today and we need to be realistic about our size, honest about our shape and aware of what we can do to achieve optimum health.

Myth #2: Size 2 Women have "thin genes."

The misconception that thin women are genetically different, preordained by nature to be at their ideal weight is simply NOT true. Lifestyle choices make the difference. I've worked with hundreds of women who used to believe that it was their genetic destiny to be overweight, only to be proven wrong! Once they changed their eating and exercise habits they realized that they too could be one of those "naturally thin" women. All it takes is the willingness to exercise 40 – 60 minutes 5 days a week and eat a nutritious, calorie conscious diet. See, it's really just NATURAL!

We each have a unique body. Science is proving that some of us have a stronger propensity towards gaining weight while others not. But, the fact remains that a healthy active lifestyle with targeted and consistent exercise, is the key to overcoming this genetic propensity to gain weight through body shaping and sculpting. We can change the way our bodies look on the outside and how efficient they are on the inside. Anyone can lose weight. If being overweight was the direct result of genetics, then weight loss would not be possible for those genetically predisposed to be obese. Instead, we know that, although some individuals burn calories less efficiently due to metabolic differences, obesity can still be reversed with good diet and adequate exercise. While it's probably true that not everyone can or should be an actual size 2, we can't blame heredity for the fact that we can barely fit into a size 22!

> *"I'm a size 2 and I'm very conscious of my health as my family history on both parents' sides' includes diabetes, heart disease and cancer. I ran my first ½ marathon the year before last and am registered to run it again. I maintain my weight through running and other aerobic exercise and weight training.*
>
> *Being African-American and small is nearly an oxymoron, it seems. I am always being asked whether I am stressed or that I need to eat. So there's definitely a pressure in my culture to be a certain size. I do enjoy all of the foods not good for me, but I don't eat them on a regular basis." - Margo Williams Handy*

Myth #3: Thin = Healthy.

Just because she looks hot in her jeans doesn't make her the picture of health. Hey, she may be on her 3rd nonfat, soy, 3-spelenda latte of the day and looking forward to a dinner of French Fries. Her fitness regime could consist of text messaging and channel surfing. This woman can be classified as what I call "Skinny Fat." "Skinny Fat" women usually look great until you ask them to climb a flight of stairs or carry a grocery bag. They don't eat healthy or exercise regularly to keep that lean frame. They subsist on limited amounts of junk food and other bad habits which can include such dangerous practices as smoking tobacco to curb their appetite. They may look skinny, but their true % of body fat is high, for example a 30-year-old women weighing 110 lbs. should have a body fat percentage of between 16-22%. A" skinny fat" women could weigh 110 lbs. but have a body fat percentage of 32! They may look thin, but the woman with the 32% body fat is at risk for all the diseases associated with being obese.

We're all aware of serious psychological eating disorders, such as Bulimia and Anorexia. We know that these conditions have grave consequences and damage the body despite the fact that many of those suffering may just look "thin." But, did you know that there is now another category for the thin and unhealthy. Have you heard of Drunkorexia? Yes, Drunkorexia! Drunkorexics severely limit their calories in order to binge on alcohol. Like anorexia and bulimia, drunkorexia stems from the combination of a propensity toward alcoholism in conjunction with a preoccupation with weight and a desire to be excessively thin.

It's imperative that we recognize the difference between healthy weight loss and a life threatening disorder. Being thin is not always healthy and definitely not always happy if the journey to get there is not based upon the pursuit of long term health.

Myth #4: Others want you to get fit.

You've been working out, eating healthy, looking and feeling great; so why all the dirty looks? "Wow, you look great. How much weight have you lost?" You may expect to hear this instead of "Come on, you can have a little piece of cake." Your friends, family and coworkers can actually have a negative influence on your weight loss and health goals. Feeling threatened and jealous by your weight loss often leads to snide remarks, "You're always going to the gym," "I tried that diet and it didn't work."

Don't expect everyone to support you. When the "eating relationship" you may have shared with friends and family before embarking on your transformative health path ends, it's up to you to be honest and firm about your new lifestyle. Statistics show that obesity is contagious. If you have a friend who becomes obese, your chances of becoming obese increase by 57%, as cited by Nicholas A. Christakis, M.D., Ph.D., M.P.H., and James H. Fowler, Ph.D., *The New England Journal of Medicine*, July 2007. So, although support is always welcome and helpful, the true motivation to achieve your goals must ultimately come from within.

Myth #5: It's too expensive to eat healthy.

The fast food dollar menu looks like a bargain to many, but when you take into consideration the long term cost on your health, there is nothing cheap about it. The best way to eat healthy and stick to your budget is to buy foods in their least processed form, prepare them yourself, and plan ahead. Sounds like a lot more work than the drive through, but the satisfaction you receive from eating real food rather than a concoction of genetically modified processed crap is worth the effort.

Don't make excuses, make a plan to find your local farmers market, start cooking at home and reap the many benefits of better health, a smaller waistline and not a thinner wallet.

Myth #6: You'll never be a Size 2 after having a baby.

Celebrities like; Jessica Alba, Gwyneth Paltrow and Jennifer Garner make it look ridiculously easy to regain their pre-pregnancy physiques. But the bottom line is that these women work out (hard) and eat right to lose the baby weight. Yes, they have access to personal chiefs, around the clock nannies and personal trainers, but you can do it too (without the celebrity perks) by following these strategies[2]:

---

[2] Always consult your doctor about the exercise plan that is safe for you during pregnancy. The American College of Obstetricians and Gynecologists recommends resuming your pre-

✓ Reach a healthy weight before becoming pregnant. If you haven't been exercising, start before you conceive so that you can continue light to moderate exercise during your pregnancy.

✓ Cardio & Resistance Workouts: 30-55 minutes 3-5 days per week.

"When you're 35, you either starve yourself or you eat and you do serious cardio," Paltrow said on *OPRAH* 2008

✓ Eat highly nutritious, calorie balanced meals and snacks. Start with the *Size 2* 21-Day Plan

"It took me a long, long time. I just wasn't that motivated. I wanted to play with her. Then I got on the treadmill, stopped stuffing my face and lost the weight. I cut out croissants, bagels and muffins – all the good stuff and went back to having a salad once a day and protein. "Jennifer Garner PEOPLE Magazine 2007

✓ Breastfeeding can help women burn an extra 500 to 600 calories a day.

"I lost the tummy just breastfeeding, and I do cardio on my own. I'm doing it slow." Jessica Alba OK Magazine 2008

Now, while we're on the subject of celebrities and diets, let's examine some that don't work!

---

pregnancy routine based on your personal physical capability. Always ask your doctor when it is safe for you to begin an exercise program.

Why 'Celebrity Diets' Don't Work

Although the *Size 2 for Life* program stresses the benefits of a healthy slim body we also emphasize the distinction between healthy vs. extreme. The pressure for celebrities to have perfect bodies often leads to unhealthy and extreme dieting. It's unfortunate that many stick-thin actresses claim to eat healthy diets and exercise with their trainers regularly. I find that impossible to believe. Subsisting on a diet of caffeine, nicotine, and an occasional calorie does not provide enough energy for basic bodily functions, let alone exercise.

Although we regard a frame adjusted[3] size 2 as ideal for the majority of women, many women I've trained get discouraged that they can't attain the size 0 that they see on TV or in magazines. They often feel "fat," although they are at an ideal weight, with perfect body composition, are exercising regularly, and are eating a nutritious diet. It's important to understand that just because someone looks incredibly thin; it doesn't mean they're lean or healthy. Extreme dieters often lose lean muscle, altering their body composition and increasing their body fat percentage. Even though they have a low body weight, they are "Skinny Fat." It is important to question images in the media and to remember health, energy, and happiness are not found in extreme thinness.

Many celebrities suffer from eating disorders or have adopted disordered eating behaviors to maintain such low body weights.

Here's a look at the dangerous, difficult and diligent disorders of celebrity weight loss.

The Dangerous

Master Cleanse
The "Master Cleanse" is a fast that requires subsisting for 10 or more days solely on fresh-squeezed lemon juice, cayenne pepper, maple syrup, and water.

Beyoncé Knowles

Announced that she had lost 20 pounds on the fast to prepare for her starring role in the film *Dreamgirls*.

"I lived on water, cayenne pepper, and maple syrup for 14 days. It was tough; everyone was eating and I was dying." – Beyoncé Knowles on *Oprah*, 2006

The One Meal Per Day Plan

---

[3] See section on adjusting for frame size

Liz Hurley

Reportedly lost post baby weight with the Caveman Diet. This diet relies on the theory that we don't need three meals a day. She ate just one meal a day and never mixed proteins with carbohydrates.

Victoria Beckham

Reportedly eats one meal a day, consisting of steamed fish, vegetables, and salad, in order to maintain her painfully thin figure.

Mariah Carey

Purple Food Diet

Reportedly, three days a week she eats nothing but grapes, plums, beetroots, and other purple-hued foods.

Sarah Michelle Gellar

Cabbage Soup Diet

Reportedly ate cabbage soup for seven days, along with fruit, vegetables, fish, and chicken. Sarah Michelle claimed to lose 30 lbs.

The Smoking Weight Loss Plan?

We all know better – smoking kills. Unfortunately, smoking is also viewed as an appetite suppressant, and many desperate to lose weight will do anything – including risk their health – to do so.

Who "Lights Up to Lighten Up"

- Jennifer Aniston
- Drew Barrymore
- Neve Campbell
- Sheryl Crow
- Claire Danes
- Johnny Depp
- Cameron Diaz
- Shannon Daugherty
- Minnie Driver
- Colin Farrell
- Lindsay Lohan
- Courtney Love
- Kate Moss
- Sarah Jessica Parker
- Michelle Pfiefer
- Joaquin Phoenix

- Christina Ricci

The Difficult

THE RAW FOOD DIET
Followers of the Raw Food Diet eat only uncooked food.

- Alicia Silverstone
- Carol Alt
- Demi Moore
- Woody Harrelson
- Sting
- Seal
- Uma Thurman

THE MACROBIOTIC DIET
The Macrobiotic Diet includes whole grains such as rice and quinoa, fresh vegetables and fruits, seaweeds, and fermented foods such as soy. Followers avoid processed foods.

- Madonna
- Courtney Love
- Gwyneth Paltrow

The Diligent Zone Followers

Barry Sears invented the Zone Diet. It advises eating a specific ratio of carbohydrates, protein, and fats: specifically 40 percent: 30 percent: 30 percent. Ideally, every meal and snack should provide 40 percent of calories from carbohydrate, 30 percent from protein, and 30 percent from fat. This is what some Zone fans call the 40:30:30 plan.

- Jennifer Aniston
- Sandra Bullock
- Cindy Crawford
- Sarah Jessica Parker
- Brad Pitt
- Rene Zelleweger

Why Can't I Look Like That?
You Can...Get Photoshop

It's an illusion – the flawlessness skin, perfect hair, flat stomachs, fuller breasts, pumped lips, and toned muscles. These robotic magazine images often perpetuate unrealistic ideals. Although we know that magazine covers and photos are retouched, the images still leave many feeling hopeless and defeated. I've had clients bring me images of celebrity body parts they cut out of magazines, hoping to achieve the jiggle-free arms or flat stomach. The focus on perfection is counterproductive; remember, an entire team of hair, makeup, lighting, and retouching professionals were required to create that photograph.

Happily, there is a backlash to all of this retouching. Some celebrities like Kate Winslet don't want their images drastically altered. Advertising campaigns, like DOVE, are emphasizing "real women," and there are now a new generation of fitness magazines, which are using true life "reader models," and thus creating healthier, more realistic role models.

Eating Disorders

Many celebrities suffer from eating disorders or have adopted disordered eating behaviors to maintain such low body weights.

Anorexia and Bulimia

Anorexia nervosa is a complex psychological eating disorder. There are new rumors every week about which celebrities are anorexic. Is she or isn't she…? Being skinny does not necessarily imply that one has anorexia. Anorexia is an eating disorder where people literally starve themselves. It usually begins in young people around the onset of puberty. People suffering from anorexia are very skinny, but are convinced that they are overweight. Since they believe they are overweight, they refuse to eat, often developing serious medical complications that sometimes result in death.

Bulimia nervosa is a psychological condition in which a person engages in binge eating followed by intentional purging. Purging can take the form of vomiting, the use of laxatives, diuretics or other medication, or excessive exercise. Today eating disorders constitute a major health concern. According to the National Eating Disorders Organization, between 5 million and 10 million girls and women, and 2 million boys and men have some type of eating disorder. As many as 15 percent of the men and women, boys and girls, who are diagnosed as having anorexia nervosa will die from that disorder. An amazing 1 out of 5 college-aged women are engaging in some form of bulimic behavior (binging and purging).

If you think you may suffer from anorexia or bulimia, please get the help you need.

http://www.nationaleatingdisorders.org

Some well-known actresses have confirmed their struggles with anorexia and bulimia, others vehemently deny the accusations that they have an eating disorder.

Jamie-Lynn DiScala, actress

Battled severe anorexia and "exercise bulimia" in high school, wrote a book about it (2002's *Wise Girl*), and is now a spokeswoman for the National Eating Disorders Association.

"I was fortunate enough in that I could afford therapists, psychiatrists and nutritionists." *New York Post*

Calista Flockhart, actress

The former *Ally McBeal* star told *People* in 1988:

"I'm not too thin. Am I anorexic? I guess my answer would have to be no."

Later she admitted that she struggled with anorexia while filming the show.

"I started under-eating, over-exercising, pushing myself too hard and brutalizing my immune system."

Courtney Thorne-Smith, actress

Battled an eating disorder and developed anorexia due to the pressure to be thin. Her slide into anorexia led her to quit the television show *Ally Mc Beal*. "The amount of time I spent thinking about food and being upset about my body was insane.'' *People*

Portia de Rossi, actress

Admitted to *Vogue* magazine that she struggled with anorexia while starring on the hit show *Ally McBeal*.

"I've often wondered if I wasn't on that show if [anorexia] may not have happened. I didn't really know at that point what it was like to be a celebrity, and the only people I knew at the time who had a similar experience were these women whom I worked with. They became my role models."

Tracey Gold, actress

Sought treatment for anorexia. "All life meant was losing weight, counting calories." *People*, 1994

Christina Ricci, actress

"I did get all my tips from a Tracey Gold Lifetime movie on anorexia. It taught me what to do." *Jane*, 2002

Billy Bob Thornton, actor

"Frankly, for a while there, I think I had a little mental problem," said Thornton, who lost 59 pounds. "I got anorexic; of course I denied it to my girlfriend and everyone else who said I had an eating disorder." *LA Daily News*, 1998

Victoria Beckham (Posh Spice), singer

"I was very obsessed. I mean, I could tell you the fat content and the calorie content in absolutely anything. I was never anorexic, I was never bulimic, but I was probably very close to it." ABC's *20/20*, 2003

Ashlee Simpson, singer

"I was around a lot of girls with eating disorders, and I actually had a minor one myself. It was about six months of not eating too much at all." *Cosmopolitan*, 2005

Mary-Kate Olsen

Mary-Kate Olsen has sought treatment for anorexia.

Paula Abdul

Battled bulimia and sought treatment in 1994. She is now a spokesperson for the National Eating Disorder Association (NEDA).

Kristen Haglund

Miss America, 2008, was diagnosed with anorexia in 2005. She now works to raise awareness of eating disorders.

Be sure to seek professional help if you think you may be suffering from an eating disorder.

> *I applaud your effort to communicate about healthy weight maintenance. I have a good friend who went through anorexia when we were in college and it was absolutely devastating for her and all of us who supported her during the ordeal. I hate to see the Hollywood types and models falling into that trap because it's a job requirement to be thinner than their bodies are meant to be... I'm 5'6 ½ tall, 125 lbs and a size 2 the healthy way." - Tracy Shilobrit*

"ALLI" – Oops!

Without going into great detail, let me just say that trying to lose weight through medicinal means such as stimulants, hormones, steroids, and the latest craze of (essentially) purgatives are doomed to failure.

The distributor, Glaxo-Smith-Kline, along with their compliant physician disciples would have you believe that Alli is designed to be used by people who already have a low caloric intake of fat, to inhibit an additional percentage of fat from being absorbed, and thus, the side effects should be minimal. They advertise that people who are not able to limit their fat intake should not take Alli, due to its very unpleasant side effect of uncontrollable diarrhea.

Well, the fact is: People with low consumption of fat don't need Alli at all. What the manufactures don't tell you is that the real target consumers are actually the ones who can't limit their intake of fat and want a fast, simple, and artificial means of circumventing the issue. Of course, these are exactly the people who will have the highest incidence of the very unpleasant side effect (oops!), and shouldn't be taking the medication in the first place. Furthermore, the fear of unpleasant side effects can also be a strong deterrent to taking part in the increased activities that are so essential to weight loss, changing your mindset and establishing a healthy lifestyle. We ask that our readers do not utilize Alli as an addition to the *Size 2 for Life* program.

Size 2 Do's & Don'ts

Do's

Do make a plan.
Work out a strategy that will motivate you to change the habits and attitudes that may have undermined your past efforts to lose weight.

- Choose a definite start date.
- Plan how often and how long you'll exercise.
- Make your daily exercise a priority on your schedule.
- Determine a realistic eating plan and stick to it.
- Set small goals.

Remember that you're in this for the long haul. You're making lifestyle changes, and the goals you've written down are your first baby steps in that direction.

Do create a mantra.
Find a short phrase or word that empowers you to achieve your goal. A friend of mine always says "A healthy plate means my ideal weight." Have fun with it. Be silly or serious and just find something that resonates with you. Examples: "I am healthy, happy and feel great;" "I am sleek, slim and sexy;" or, "I am full of abundant health and energy."

Do create an automatic response.
It takes discipline to say "no" time and again when someone offers you unhealthy food or unhealthy choices. Create an automatic response, something you'll say when someone offers you something you shouldn't eat or an activity that takes you away from your healthy lifestyle.

Do change your lifestyle.
Eliminate "empty" calories and increase your physical activity! This is the formula for lifelong health and fitness!

Do Exercise.
Performing daily exercise is probably the single most important predictor of whether you'll succeed at long term weight loss and weight loss maintenance. In order for exercise to be helpful in weight loss you should schedule your sessions like any other important commitment.

Do keep a food journal.
Keep track of everything you eat and drink. This is the best way to insure your success. Yes, it does take a few minutes every day, but for this small investment of time you'll be empowered to make better choices. You'll become involved with your progress and cognizant of where your difficulties lie. It's a proven strategy. Give it a try, stick to it, and

write your way to size 2. Use your new awareness to keep you on track and focused on your goals. Every time you eat something, record the following information in your journal:

- Time of day
- Food eaten and portion size
- Your mood
- Your hunger level and satisfaction level after eating
- Where you're eating

Do get enough sleep.
Aim to get at least 7 hours of sleep per night. Research has shown that people deprived of sleep had lower levels of the hormones that control appetite. When we're tired we crave more sugar and refined carbohydrates, both of which can put on extra pounds.

Do drink water.
Increasing water consumption helps regulate metabolism, so try drinking a glass before meals and snacks. Mix in some fiber to help fill you up before the meal.

Do eat (a healthy) breakfast every day.
According to the National Weight Control Registry, 78% of people who've lost over 30 pounds and more importantly have kept the weight off for more than a year, eat breakfast daily.

Do get support.
A big key in long-term weight control comes from receiving encouragement and support from others. Tell friends, family and co-workers that you are committed to living a healthier lifestyle.

Do monitor your progress.
Weigh yourself every week. Research has shown that people who have been successful with long-term weight loss keep track of their weight weekly. Keeping track of your progress helps you stay committed and keeps you from sliding back to old habits.

Do read labels.
Carefully read the labels of the foods you eat. Look at the calories in one serving, the grams of fat, sodium, sugar and fiber. Many food items are cleverly packaged so that a consumer thinks they're eating a single serving, but are actually ingesting two or more.

Do stay on track.
There will be days when you don't feel like working out, slip from eating right, or lack motivation. Small setbacks are part of life. Learn from your past successes and failures. Move on and learn, so that next time you'll make healthier choices toward positive goals.

Do celebrate your successes!

Every time you drop 5 lbs., lose an inch, feel stronger during your workout session or have more energy, celebrate! Do something you enjoy and thank yourself for all of your positive efforts. Remember you're getting healthier, stronger and closer to reaching your goal.

Don'ts

Don't Make Excuses.

"I'll start Monday." This familiar refrain is uttered all too often after a weekend of poor lifestyle choices. Make the commitment to yourself to be free of excuses that leave you feeling unmotivated and lacking discipline. Understand your time and physical limitations from the outset and work within them.

Don't eat late.

This can be one of the toughest things not to do, but eating late can undo all the healthy choices and actions you've achieved throughout the day. If at all possible, set an eating "cut off" time, ideally more than 3 hours before you get to bed and stick to it. In the meal section we've provided some healthy, low calorie snacks for those of you who simply can't do this, but you're journey to size 2 will be greatly accelerated if you can adhere to this rule.

Don't be unrealistic.

If you want to lose 50 pounds and you give yourself a 30 day timeframe to do it you're setting yourself up to fail. Realize that you need to be consistent, clear and realistic in the timeframe it'll take for you to achieve your goal.

Don't wait longer than 3 hours between eating.

Even a small snack can save you from overeating. If you wait too long between eating it's more difficult to control overeating at the next meal. Also, make sure you plan ahead by preparing your snacks in advance.

Don't buy junk.

Clean out your cupboards! Throw away the temptation to eat unhealthy foods. Get rid of anything that's not on your meal plan. Take a large bag and donate the food to a local shelter or just toss the junk food. If you have unhealthy options in your home you're sabotaging your success.

Don't eat out (as often).

Not only will you save some money, you'll also save on calories. It's possible to make healthy selections at restaurants, but the portions are usually larger and it's more difficult to know how many calories you're consuming. If you are eating out, opt for the low fat protein entrée along with some steamed vegetables. Don't order the starches (potatoes, bread, etc) and fatty sides (butter, margarine, dressings) and request that the waiter not bring them at all. Replace eating out and experiment with new healthier ways to cook at home.

Don't "clean your plate!"
No offense to our wonderful mothers, but don't take their advice. Being a "plate cleaner" is not a good thing. That doesn't mean we have to waste food. Sharing a meal is a great option if you're eating in a restaurant. Otherwise, get in the habit of dividing your food in half and asking for a take home bag. While living in Japan I learned the expression, "hara hachi bu," meaning eat until you are 80% full. The Japanese have perfected this technique and enjoy their meals without overeating.

Don't self-sabotage.
Your thoughts can be defeating. "I've already messed up on my meal plan, so it doesn't matter if I eat a second piece of cake." Negative thoughts like these, often-called negative self-talk, may sabotage your good intentions.

Don't consume alcohol!
Alcohol is not going to help in any area of a reduced caloric way of eating. One ounce of alcohol contains anywhere from 90 to 130 calories (7 calories per gram) and it lowers inhibitions, which may lead you to binge if you imbibe. Your best bet? Steer clear of drinking alcohol, including wine and beer, except on rare occasions. Opt for water, iced tea or fruit juices instead.

Don't eat in front of the television or in the car.
Eating while you watch the TV or driving often leads to unconscious overeating. Make your meal time special. As you become more mindful while you eat you'll not only enjoy the food you eat more, you'll also feel satisfied and satiated. Enjoy your meals. Be mindful and be grateful.

Don't give up!
We all have occasional setbacks, but instead of giving up, simply start fresh the next day. Remember that you're planning to change your life. It won't happen all at once, but stick to your new healthy lifestyle and the results will be lifelong!

Don't be sweet!

When I work with clients and have them keep food logs I'm amazed at the amounts of sugar that most women consume. I too was once a "sugar addict" and I can tell you from firsthand experience sugar is a drug. I would get headaches and so irritable until I had my fix and then I'd be happy and high - until the crash. Be honest, how often do you plan your day around your "treat?" We laugh about having to have our chocolate fix or ice cream to treat our PMS, but sugar actually makes it all worse. There is no recommended daily allowance of sugar, why? Because you should NOT eat it! Sugar is bad for you, you know this. There is a ton of scientific research that highlights all the reasons not to eat it, including: raises risk of developing diabetes, lowers your immune system, and contributes to weight gain and many other unpleasant effects on your health. All of which stand in your way of achieving the joys of that incredible size 2!

Now stop patting yourself on the back because you only use artificial sweeteners. After extensive research as well as personal observations I can tell you that if healthy living, weight loss and fitness are your goals, you should avoid artificial sweeteners and be aware of their effect on your body. *You* control what *you* put in your body and therefore *you* should take the time to know what you're ingesting.

Read the labels! Artificial sweeteners are a huge part of the American diet. These diet demons are contained in candy, packaged food and gum, and are also found in abundance in foods labeled low-calorie or diet. Here are the five FDA approved artificial sweeteners:

- Saccharin
- Aspartame
- Sucralose (known as *Splenda*, it is NOT a natural sweetener!)
- Acesulphame
- Neotame

Here are some of the potential side effects that have been reported from the use of these chemicals:

- Increased hunger levels leading to increased caloric intake!
- Resistance to insulin that could lead to major health problems!
- Potential disruption of brain chemistry leading to seizure risk and depression!
- Cancer!
- Hair loss!
- Dementia!

Personally I don't want to ingest chemicals and you also have the choice not to. I encourage my clients to avoid artificial sweeteners, sugar and high fructose corn syrup - all of it! As you'll see later in the book, the first 5 days of the *Size 2 for Life Diet & Fitness Program* are specifically designed to help you shake the sugar addiction while launching you on your journey to size 2.

The Size 2 for Life Diet & Fitness Program

The Basics

First

Get cleared by your doctor. The worst thing you can do is hurt yourself, so before you start any exercise program make sure you get a complete checkup from your doctor, including an evaluation of your spine, knees, and hips. I would also advise a diagnostic evaluation by a cardiologist, particularly if you are over 40 or if there is any history of cardiovascular disease in your family.

Second

Understand your limitations and start off slowly. The worst thing you can do is injure yourself – SO DON'T DO IT. The last thing you need is to be laid up with an injury, depressed, and eating chips and guacamole.

It's normal to have a slight amount of tightness in your muscles when starting an exercise program. If you're tight with pain the day after, then you overdid it, and you need to cut back at least 50% on the intensity (not duration) of your program.

Pep Talk Time! Let's Make a Plan!

In order to reach your health and fitness goals, you must have a road map to follow.

Step One

Start by asking yourself how much total weight you want to lose? To shrink a size you need to lose approximately 10 - 15 lbs. For example: if you're a size 10 you'll probably need to lose at least 30 lbs to attain a size 2. Wait! Don't let these numbers discourage you; just 10 lbs loss will bring you to a size 8 and just another 10 and you're already down to a very impressive size 6. Think of your journey in these terms and you'll be astounded how quickly you get to that 2.

Next calculate your frame size. This is important because women with a larger frame size may actually look emaciated as an actual size 2. These women would not be healthy at a size 2 but would look incredible as what we call a "frame adjusted" size 2. Good examples might be Brooke Shields, Halle Berry and Heidi Klum.

What size is your frame?

If you are left-handed, extend your right arm. If you are right-handed, extend your left arm. With your free hand, wrap your thumb and middle finger around your extended wrist. Be sure to wrap it around the joint section of your wrist – very close to the base of your hand.

Small Frame: If your middle finger and thumb overlap, you have a small frame.

Medium Frame: If your middle finger and thumb touch, you have a medium frame.

Large Frame: If your middle finger and thumb do not meet, you have a large frame.

A more precise estimate of frame size can be obtained with a tape measurement of your non-dominant wrist. Measure your wrist at the wrist joint. Use the following lists to find your frame size.

For women less than 5'2" in height:
- Small = wrist size less than 5.5"
- Medium = wrist size 5.5" to 5.75"
- Large = wrist size over 5.75"

For women with height between 5'2"and 5' 5"
- Small = wrist size less than 6"
- Medium = wrist size 6" to 6.25"
- Large = wrist size over 6.25"

For women with a height over 5' 5"
- Small = wrist size less than 6.25"
- Medium = wrist size 6.25" to 6.5"
- Large = wrist size over 6.5"

The following table will give you your target waist and hip sizes and help you understand where you currently stand. Notice that we exclude bust size because, let's face it ladies, that's a totally different matter!

TARGET SIZE CHART

Pant Size	0	2	4	6	8	10	12	14	16	18	20
Waist (inches)	23	24	25	26	27	28	30	31	33	35	37
Hip (inches)	34	35	36	37	38	39	40	42	43	45	47

Frame adjusted target sizes

Vanity Sizing

As mentioned previously in our section on Size 2 Myths, since the 1950's, manufacturers have been increasing the measurements. If you look at a sewing pattern from the 1950's a size 12 was: Bust 32 Waist: 26 ½ Hip 36. Today that is a size 4. Most size 4 women I know would be horrified to know that in the 50's they would have been buying size 12 jeans. It's just a silly number and it shouldn't matter, but we need to be clear that the size may be appealing more to our vanity than reality. It's clear that the clothing manufacturers understand the psychology of women and know that we'll pay more to wear the size 2, and in general, the more you pay the smaller size you'll wear. Designer labels are usually 2 sizes larger than the label says, that's what is known as "vanity sizing".

I know a celebrity personal shopper and she confided that she has to cut out the original size label and replace it with a smaller size to satisfy her client. I guess that's one way to always be a size 2.

Weight Loss Pace:

Now that you know your target weight and frame size, you need to set a reasonable weight loss pace for yourself. You can base your own pace on any number of factors, including the results of the fitness assessment we offer later on in this chapter, but a great place to start would be the general recommendations from the American College of Sports Medicine, which are one to two pounds per week.

Step Two - Eating Plan

First, look at your eating habits, such as when you eat, what you eat, how much you eat, where you eat, and how often you eat. If you feel out of control, start by keeping a journal and write down everything you eat. Seeing it on paper helps put the numbers in perspective and will help you gain control.

Plan all of your meals. Yes, it's a lot of work at first, but the extra effort really creates the discipline you need to stick with it long-term. Get on track by shopping only with a list. Get yourself on an eating schedule that has you eating small, balanced meals or snacks every two to three hours.

Finding the Best Diet for YOU

A central message of this book is that YOU can be your best fitness trainer. You know your body better than anyone. You should care about your body and health more than anyone. It has been said our bodies are our curriculum for life. We can listen to and learn from our bodies to achieve invigorating health to enjoy all areas of our lives.

It's similar to the notion that you must be your own best money manager. You may be able to find professionals to help you in this area, consultants and interested family members too, but at the end of the day, you need to know the numbers to make sure your interests are being looked after.

The more you know about your own body, the way it works, what makes it feel good, how it is a unique gift, the more empowered you will be in all areas of your life. This means you have to be keenly aware of what you put in your body and how nutrition is a key component to your health.

> *"I've lived as a size four for years after a lifetime of varying between sizes 6 and 12. The difference, which I know supports me for life, is that I listen to my intuition now. I am the one who best knows what my body needs and wants, and I respond to it."* - Karen L. Garvey, Bridging the Realms, www.TheAnswersUnlimited.com

When I work with clients and have them keep daily food logs, not only to keep track of calories, but also to increase their awareness of how certain foods affect how they feel. It is exciting to realize that a simple food allergy may be the cause of your extra stomach bloating or a daily headache can be eliminating by avoiding certain foods or additives. I have learned from my clients and seen firsthand how powerful simple changes can greatly improve well-being and weight loss.

We need to be conscious of how food affects us, the best way to figure out if you are having negative reactions to foods is to experiment and keep a log of how you feel if you eliminate certain foods and additives. For example, I was working with a woman who was motivated to lose weight for her wedding. She was experiencing terrible headaches every day, stress seemed to be a logical conclusion, but after looking at her food logs I noticed that she was consuming over ten packets of artificial sweetener per day. She had never used artificial sweetener prior to her wedding weight loss program. I have always been an advocate of a clean, chemical free diet full of organic fruits and vegetables, so I recommend she eliminate the artificial sweeteners and in less than a week she was free of her headaches.

Your body is always talking to you so listen and observe how you feel after eating. You control what you put in your body and therefore you should take the time of knowing what you are ingesting. Many trainers will not go over this with you and some trainers even endorse diets products that are full of chemicals simply because they are low in calories. I will share information with you here that I have learned, but it is my hope that you learn more on your own and continue listening to your body.

What type of diet will give you the greatest amount of energy, health and help you maintain your ideal weight? The answer is different for each of us. Each one of us needs to experiment to find the "right" diet. I've trained people who feel best on high protein diets others who swear by raw food diets and many who maintain their ideal weight by watching their portions while enjoying a variety of foods.

If you are open to trying new ways of eating, go for it! Try out a vegetarian: someone who eats no animals (no cows, pigs, chickens, fish, etc.); vegan: eats no animal products (no animals, dairy, eggs, etc.); or a raw "foodist": who eats only raw foods (no heating above 120°).

If you choose to experiment with a new way of eating pay close attention to how you feel, you may be surprised at an increase in your energy as you eliminate processed foods.

Follow these basic guidelines with any type of diet plan you choose:

> Eat a wide variety of whole foods. Foods that are in their natural form with the least possible processing.

> Eat sufficient, high quality low-fat proteins.

> Try to consume 1-cup fresh fruit and 4-6 cups fresh vegetables daily.

> Be moderate with your starch intake (carbohydrates) bread, rice, corn breads and pastas).

> Reduce animal fats and eliminate hydrogenated and processed oils. Eliminate processed snack foods (chips, cookies, crackers, cakes...)

Possible Food Allergies

> Artificial Colors
> Artificial Sweeteners
> Beer
> Chocolate
> Coffee
> Cane Sugar
> Dairy Products
> Eggs
> Gluten (a protein found in wheat, rye, barley, and oats)
> Legumes
> MSG (Monosodium glutamate, a common food additive)
> Nightshades (tomatoes, potatoes, eggplant, peppers, tobacco)
> Nuts (all kinds)
> Seeds
> Strawberries
> Wheat
> Yeast

"I'm a woman who spent 20 years 15-20 pounds overweight. I ate for emotional reasons and didn't exercise consistently. It took a long time, but I finally figured things out and learned how to eat again, got serious about exercising, and slowly lost weight to where I have been a size 4 (actually the shorts I'm wearing as I type this

are a size 2) for the past eight years. I love to hike and run, and do some sort of exercise (but not to any extremes) almost every day.

It's funny, a woman who I just met referred to me as "skinny" and that still doesn't register with me… I might appear that way, but I'm actually quite muscular and medium-framed. I don't think I'll ever be skinny, but I'm pretty happy where I am, finally." - Krista Van Lewen

Step Three - Exercise Plan

Start out slow; you don't want to burn yourself out after the first week. If you aren't currently working out, aim for two or three sessions per week. Once you feel comfortable with three sessions, keep adding every two weeks until you're exercising five days a week.

Keep in mind that the four important components of your workout program are:

- Frequency
- Duration
- Intensity
- Type (Mode)

Frequency of Exercise

The first component of cardiovascular exercise is frequency of the exercise, which refers to the number of exercise sessions per week. To improve both cardiovascular fitness and to decrease body fat or maintain body fat at optimum levels, you should do cardiovascular exercise at least three days a week. The American College of Sports Medicine recommends three to five days a week for most cardiovascular programs. We would ultimately like to see you work your way up to daily if possible. Those of you who are very out of shape and/or who are overweight and doing weight-bearing cardiovascular exercise, such as an aerobics class or jogging, might want to have at least 36–48 hours of rest between workouts in order to prevent an injury and to promote adequate bone and joint stress recovery.

Duration of Exercise

The second component of cardiovascular exercise is the duration, which refers to the time you've spent exercising. The cardiovascular session, not including the warm up and cool down, should vary from 30–60 minutes to gain significant cardio-respiratory and fat-burning benefits.

It is important that you gradually increase the duration before you increase the intensity. For example, when beginning a walking program, be more concerned with increasing the number of minutes of the exercise session before you increase the intensity by increasing your speed or by walking hilly terrain.

Types of Exercise (Mode)

Aerobic Exercise – Cardiovascular Strength Training – Muscular Strength and Endurance Exercise – Flexibility – Stretching and Warm-up Exercises

Intensity (How Hard You Are Working Out)

One of the most common mistakes new exercisers make is in not measuring exercise intensity. You might make the mistake of working too hard (which can lead to injury and burnout), or not working hard enough (which can lead to frustration from lack of results).

There are different ways to measure your intensity. The most common ways are:

- **Target Heart Rate**

- **Rate of Perceived Exertion (RPE)** – how easily can you speak while you're exercising? *See section "alternative to target heart rates."*

Fitness Assessment

If you belong to a gym that offers a free introductory fitness assessment you might want to opt for it to help determine your current fitness level. Although many clients opt not to do the fitness assessment, I recommend it as a good way to establish your baseline and help track your progress. But you can do all the basic assessments on your own – so grab a stopwatch and get ready.

Before starting or continuing any exercise program, ask yourself some basic questions:

1. What is my current level of fitness and physical activity?

2. What are my fitness goals?

3. What is my daily resting heart rate?

4. What is my maximum heart rate?

For a beginning exerciser, a sensible goal is to improve overall health and to adapt to a more active, energetic lifestyle. Beginners should monitor their heart rate and train aerobically (80% of maximum or below) for at least the first three months of their program. Heart rate zones may be determined by using the 220 or 226 minus age formula. More experienced exercisers may have goals like performance improvement or body composition changes. These entail designing an annual calendar of workout according to heart rate guidelines, and regular performance testing to monitor overtraining and improvement.

According to the American Medical Association, your maximum heart rate is approximately 220 minus your age. Your target heart rate is generally between 50 and 75 percent of your maximum heart rate. This is your ideal heart rate to reach during aerobic exercise such as brisk walking or jogging.

Target Heart Rates

AHA Recommendation

Health professionals know the importance of proper pacing during exercise. To receive the benefits of physical activity, it's important not to tire too quickly. Pacing yourself is especially important if you've been inactive.

Target heart rates let you measure your initial fitness level and monitor your progress in a fitness program. This approach requires measuring your pulse periodically as you exercise and staying within 50–85 percent of your maximum heart rate. This range is called your target heart rate.

What is an alternative to target heart rates?

Some people can't measure their pulse or don't want to take their pulse when exercising. If this is true for you, try using a "conversational pace," sometimes referred to as the Rate of Perceived Exertion (RPE), to monitor your efforts during moderate activities, like walking. If you can talk and walk at the same time, you aren't working too hard. If you can sing and maintain your level of effort, you're probably not working hard enough. If you get out of breath quickly, you're probably working too hard – especially if you have to stop and catch your breath.

When should I use the target heart rate?

If you participate in more vigorous activities, like brisk walking and jogging, the "conversational pace" approach may not work. Try using the target heart rate. It works for many people, and is a good way for health professionals to monitor your progress.

The next table shows estimated target heart rates for different ages. Look for the age category closest to yours, and then read across to find your target heart rate.

Age	Target HR Zone 50–85 %	Average Maximum Heart Rate 100 %
20 years	100–170 beats per minute	200 beats per minute
25 years	98–166 beats per minute	195 beats per minute
30 years	95–162 beats per minute	190 beats per minute
35 years	93–157 beats per minute	185 beats per minute

40 years	90–153 beats per minute	180 beats per minute
45 years	88–149 beats per minute	175 beats per minute
50 years	85–145 beats per minute	170 beats per minute
55 years	83–140 beats per minute	165 beats per minute
60 years	80–136 beats per minute	160 beats per minute
65 years	78–132 beats per minute	155 beats per minute
70 years	75–128 beats per minute	150 beats per minute

Your maximum heart rate is about 220 minus your age. The figures above are averages, so use them as general guidelines.

Note: A few high blood pressure medications lower the maximum heart rate and thus the target zone rate. If you're taking such medicine, call your physician to find out if you need to use a lower target heart rate.

How should I pace myself?

When starting an exercise program, aim at the lowest part of your target zone (50 percent) during the first few weeks. Gradually build up to the higher part of your target zone (75 percent). After six months or more of regular exercise, you may be able to exercise comfortably at up to 85 percent of your maximum heart rate. However, you don't have to exercise that hard to stay in shape.

Training Zones

Healthy Heart Zone (Warm Up) — 50–60% of maximum heart rate. This is the easiest zone and probably the best zone for people just starting a fitness program. This zone has been shown to help lower body fat, blood pressure, and cholesterol. It also decreases the risk of degenerative diseases and has a low risk of injury. Of calories burned in this zone, 80% are fats!

Fitness Zone (Fat Burning) — 60-70% of maximum heart rate. This zone provides the same benefits as the healthy heart zone, but is more intense and burns more total calories. The percent of fat calories is still about in the neighborhood of 65- 80%.

Aerobic Zone (Endurance Training) — 70-80% of maximum heart rate. The aerobic zone will improve your cardiovascular and respiratory system AND increase the size and strength of your heart. This is the preferred zone if you are training for an endurance event. More calories are burned, with 50% being from fat.

The next two zones are high intensity zones. You should train in these zones only if you are in very good shape and have been cleared by a physician to do so.

Anaerobic Zone (Performance Training) — 80-90% of maximum heart rate. Benefits of this zone include an improved VO2 maximum (the highest amount of oxygen one can consume during exercise), and thus an improved cardio-respiratory system, and a higher lactate-tolerance ability, which means your endurance will improve and you'll be able to fight fatigue better. This is a high-intensity zone burning more calories, with 30% from fat.

Red Line (Maximum Effort) — 90-100% of maximum heart rate. Although this zone burns the highest number of calories/min, it is very intense. Most people can stay in this zone for only short periods.

Step Test

This test is designed to measure your cardiovascular endurance. Using a 12-inch-high bench (or a similar-sized stair in your house), step on and off for three minutes. Step up with one foot and then the other. Step down with one foot, followed by the other foot. Try to maintain a steady four-beat cycle. It's easy to maintain if you say, "Up, up, down, down." Go at a steady and consistent pace. At the end of three minutes, remain standing and immediately check your heart rate by taking your pulse for one minute.

This home step test is based on the Harvard Step Assessment. If you want to keep track of your cardiovascular improvements do this test four to six weeks after you start your exercise program and see if you have improved.

3-Minute Step Test

Age	18-25	26-35	36-45	46-55	56-65	65+
Excellent	<85	<88	<90	<94	<95	<90
Good	85-98	88-99	90-102	94-104	95-104	90-102
Above Average	99-108	100-111	103-110	105-115	105-112	103-115
Average	109-117	112-119	111-118	116-120	113-118	116-122
Below Average	118-126	120-126	119-128	121-129	119-128	123-128
Poor	127-140	127-138	129-140	130-135	129-139	129-134
Very Poor	>140	>138	>140	>135	>139	>134

Push-Up Test

How many can you do?   Women should use the "bent knee" position. To do this, kneel on the floor, hands on either side of the chest, and keep your back straight. Do as many push-ups as possible until exhaustion. Count the total number of push-ups performed. Use the chart below to find out how you rate.

Push-Up Test

Age	17-19	20-29	30-39	40-49	50-59	60-65
Excellent	>35	>36	>37	>31	>25	>23
Good	27-35	30-36	30-37	25-31	21-25	19-23
Above Average	21-27	23-29	22-30	18-24	15-20	13-18
Average	11-20	12-22	10-21	8-17	7-14	5-12
Below Average	6-10	7-11	5-9	4-7	3-6	2-4
Poor	2-5	2-6	1-4	1-3	1-2	1
Very Poor	0-1	0-1	0	0	0	0

Squat Test

How many squats can you do? Stand in front of a chair or bench with your feet at shoulder-width apart, facing away from it. Place your hands on your hips. Squat down and lightly touch the chair before standing up. A good-sized chair is one that makes your knees at right angles when you are sitting. Keep doing this until you're fatigued.

Squat Test

Age	18-25	26-35	36-45	46-55	56-65	65+
Excellent	>43	>39	>33	>27	>24	>23
Good	37-43	33-39	27-33	22-27	18-24	17-23
Above Average	33-36	29-32	23-26	18-21	13-17	14-16
Average	29-32	25-28	19-22	14-17	10-12	11-13
Below Average	25-28	21-24	15-18	10-13	7-9	5-10

| Poor | 18-24 | 13-20 | 7-14 | 5-9 | 3-6 | 2-4 |
| Very Poor | <18 | <20 | <7 | <5 | <3 | <2 |

Sit-Ups

Abdominal muscle strength and endurance are important for core stability and back support. This sit-up test measures the strength and endurance of the abdominals and hip-flexor muscles. Count how many you can do in one minute and then check the chart below for your rating.

Starting Position: Lie on a carpeted or cushioned floor, with your knees bent at approximately right angles and your feet flat on the ground. Your hands should be resting on your thighs.

Technique: Squeeze your stomach, push your back flat, and raise high enough for your hands to slide along your thighs to touch the tops of your knees. Don't pull with your neck or head, and keep your lower back on the floor. Return to the starting position.

1-Minute Sit-Up Test

Age	18-25	26-35	36-45	46-55	56-65	65+
Excellent	>43	>39	>33	>27	>24	>23
Good	37-43	33-39	27-33	22-27	18-24	17-23
Above Average	33-36	29-32	23-26	18-21	13-17	14-16
Average	29-32	25-28	19-22	14-17	10-12	11-13
Below Average	25-28	21-24	15-18	10-13	7-9	5-10
Poor	18-24	13-20	7-14	5-9	3-6	2-4
Very Poor	<18	<20	<7	<5	<3	<2

Source: adapted from Golding, et al. (1986). *The Y's way to physical fitness* (3rd ed.)

Finding Out Your Body Fat Percentage

Body Composition

Body composition is simply the ratio of lean body mass to fat body mass. Too much fat can lead to health problems like heart disease, diabetes, high cholesterol, and other serious conditions. If you keep your body fat within a reasonable level, you'll be healthier and, of course, slimmer.

For women, a body fat of 10–12% is essential, 14–20% is considered a healthy range for athletes, 21–24% is healthy for fitness, 25–31% is considered an "acceptable" range, and anything above 32% is considered obese. If you want to be a healthy, slim and sexy frame adjusted size 2, aim for a range of around 14 – 22%.

So, how do you find out what your body fat is? Here are the most popular methods for testing body composition.

Common Methods Used to Find the Fat Percentage

Calipers

This method uses calipers to measure skin fold thickness at several areas of your body.

How it works: A trainer pinches your skin at different areas and measures them with calipers. Results are plugged into a formula to determine your body fat.

Have you been pinched lately? Maybe you haven't, but you've probably heard people talking about how low their body fat is.

"Great, I have six percent body fat." Not so fast, just ask a different trainer to measure your body fat, and suddenly you have sixteen percent? The problem is there is a great deal of human error when using calipers. What would seem like a small difference in measurement can make a big difference to your overall percentage. There are many variables that affect your percentage: gender, ethnicity, fitness level, and age. The accuracy of body fat calipers is rated within 4% if you have an experienced trainer administering the test, so take it with a grain of low-sodium salt.

Hydrostatic Weighing

This is just a fancy way of saying underwater weighing. This test is one of the more accurate ones.

How it works:

You sit on a scale inside a tank of water and blow out as much air as you can. You are dunked underwater, where you blow out even more air. Since fat is lighter than water, the more fat you have, the more you'll float. The scale measures underwater weight to figure out body density. The margin of error is around 2–3%, but the accuracy depends on the amount of air you expel. You have to blow it all out or it won't be as accurate.

This is a difficult way to measure body fat, since it can be uncomfortable and even scary to be dunked underwater with no air in the old lungs. If you want to use hydrostatic weighing make sure you don't pay too much at an overpriced "Health Spa," some universities offer this test for around \$25–\$50.

Bioelectrical Impedance

I prefer this method above all others because it's quick, easy and the scales can be obtained at a variety of stores including pharmacies, department stores as well as specialty stores like *The Sharper Image* and *GNC*.

The basic principle of bioelectrical impedance is this: As you stand on the scale a signal passes from your feet; the faster the signal travels, the more muscle you have. The results are based on the fact that water conducts electricity. Fat contains almost no water, while muscle is about 70% water.

Depending on the brand of the scale, this method can be accurate within the 4% margin of error the calipers have, but the results are affected by hydration, food intake, and skin temperature. If you're dehydrated, your body fat percentage will read higher than it is. This is an easy way to test your body fat. Be sure to test it at the same time of day.

The Exercise Program

Choose Your Primary Aerobic Device

- Treadmill

- Bicycle

- Elliptical or stepper

- Do It Anywhere Cardio

- The new *Size 2 for Life - Total Fitness DVD*

Of the first three, my personal preference is the treadmill because for most people it's a device that's easy to use and has a history of success. Also, it's easy for me to get motivated to increase my pace when I combine it with some good, upbeat music and a mirror to encourage my progress. – Dr. Paulsen

For some (particularly if you are 30 or more pounds overweight), it may be preferable to begin with a bike, elliptical, stepper/climber or walking on an inclined treadmill.

The reason is that jogging can put considerable stress on the back and joints, particularly the knees – and the last thing you need is an injury!

Your choice will depend on your personal preferences and understanding of your limitations, in consultation with your physician. Whichever you choose, START OFF SLOW and ADVANCE SLOWLY. Duration is more important than intensity.

The 80/20 Rule

If you're to achieve your goal of weight loss, you need to focus on the exercises that burn calories while also toning the muscles in the process. This is exactly the opposite of what you get with a trainer. In fact, recently some well-connected "celebrity" gurus have been advocating various "cardio-free" exercise and diet programs, with as little as one hour per week of strictly resistance training. Alternatively, a trainer may tell you to get aerobic exercise on your own time. But let's be realistic – who has any more time?

I have no intention of wasting time disputing the ridiculous logic of the "cardio-free" programs. Suffice it to say that the epidemic of obesity in this country is certainly not the result of an excess of cardio-intensive exercise. In fact, there is overwhelming evidence indicating that it's most likely a direct consequence of the lack of it. Furthermore, according to a study in the "Journal of Gerontology: Medical Sciences" and reported in "The Wall Street Journal," as little as three hours of aerobic exercise per week can reverse the brain shrinkage which normally starts in a person's 40's and actually lead to regeneration of new brain cells - a phenomenon which had previously been considered impossible. Strength training and stretching had no effect whatsoever. In addition, recent studies have also demonstrated that regular aerobic exercise can actually reverse earlier radiological findings of pathology in the coronary arteries.

On the other hand, a solid resistive/toning component can be a great adjunct to an overall fitness program. As pointed out in a recent article by Dr. Mark Williams, et al., in the journal *Circulation*, some of the potential benefits may include "enhanced cardiovascular health, weight management, and prevention of disability..." The researchers further note that: "Incorporating resistance training in the training regimen can potentially improve maintenance of interest and compliance." But they also add this qualification: "Because of the extensive evidence supporting the benefits of aerobic exercise training on modulating cardiovascular risk factors...resistance training should be used as a complement to, and not a replacement for, aerobic exercise."

My personal recommendation is: Get your 70–80% aerobic exercise first, and then get your 15–20% muscle strengthening later at the gym, on your own or, if you prefer, with a trainer. – Dr. Paulsen

I find that if I do my jogging first thing in the morning, then I'm able to get in the strengthening later during the day or evening. It's far easier to find 10–20 minutes for muscle strengthening than it is to get motivated for 40–60 minutes of jogging after a hard and perhaps stressful day.

For optimum results, I recommend a program of 40–60 minutes of aerobic exercise (including the warm up) first thing in the morning, and then another 20 minutes (perhaps on an alternate device, such as a bike) in the evening, ideally along with an additional 20 minutes of strengthening. If you follow this program, in addition to the dietary recommendations, your results will be extraordinary.

Time of Day – Right Away

There are experts who would debate this point until all the celebrities get out of rehab. Some say you burn more calories at night, others say in the morning, others say some combination of both. Forget this argument. From a practical standpoint, it's all just a bunch of meaningless noise.

What you need to do is get your aerobic exercise every day, and the best way to ensure this is to do it first thing in the morning, before anything else can distract you.

I used to have to be at the clinic by 6:30 a.m. That meant getting up at 4:00 a.m. to get my exercise in. Every day I woke up, I hated myself. I fought myself, I cursed myself. But 50 lbs. later, I loved myself. You will, too. – Dr. Paulsen

So calculate 40 – 60 minutes for exercise before you do anything else and set the clock a bit earlier, if that is what it takes. And, allow no excuses from yourself. Morning exercise is your new religion.

Stretching[4]

Pay particular attention to stretching the leg muscles, especially the calf and thigh. Stretching the calf muscles is particularly important if you're jogging. Nothing will lay you up quicker than a cramped or strained gastrocnemius muscle. So make sure you stretch for at least two to five minutes before beginning your run. Make sure to use steady, slow stretching and avoid bouncing.

I often see people hop off the treadmill at the gym, rush to the shower, or jump in the car, without even a quick cool down or stretch. Great, you just ran three miles, but you may not be feeling so good tomorrow or the next day if you don't take the time to stretch out the muscles you've just worked. The keys to preventing injuries are warming up, cooling down, and stretching. - Ashley

The key to proper stretching lies in the way you perform the exercise. When you're stretching certain parts of your body, you should not feel pain. Staying relaxed is very important to stretching properly. Make sure your body is not tight. Go slow! Always stretch slowly and evenly. Hold the stretch for about fifteen seconds and release slowly, as well. Never bounce or jerk while stretching. This can cause injury as a muscle is pushed beyond its ability. All stretches should be smooth and slow. Don't forget to breathe. Flexibility exercises should be relaxing. Deep, easy, even breathing is key to relaxation. Never hold your breath while you stretch. Your shoulders, hands, and feet should be kept relaxed as you stretch.

Here are some basic stretches you should do daily.

Hamstrings: Sit on the floor with one leg straight in front of you and the other leg bent (with the sole of the foot touching the inside thigh of the outstretched leg).

---

[4] See also the "Do It Anywhere Cardio Exercises" section

Keep your back straight and lean forward from the hips.

Slide your arms forward toward your outstretched foot.

Stop when you feel a pull in the hamstring.

Hold for 15 seconds. Repeat with the other leg extended.

Hips: Lie on your back. Bend your left leg and bring it toward you.

Grasp your left knee gently with your right hand and pull it slightly down and to the right until you feel a stretch.

Turn your head to the left. Your right leg should stay flat on the floor.

Hold for 10 seconds. Repeat with the other leg.

Lower back: Lay flat on the floor with knees bent.

Cross your ankles.

Use your hands to pull your knees toward your chest.

Lift your head and shoulders off the floor until your head is approximately six inches from your knees.

Gently rock yourself back and forth in this position for 30 seconds.

Quadriceps: Bend your right leg and hold on to the ankle with your right hand.

 Hold onto a chair or stable for support if needed.

Gently pull your right heel in toward the right side of your butt.

As soon as you feel a stretch in your right quad slowly lower your right knee toward the floor, behind your left knee.

Hold for 15 seconds. Repeat with the other leg.

Calves: Stand at arm's length away from a wall, with your feet shoulder-width apart.

Slide your left foot back approximately 18 inches, keeping the knee straight and both heels flat on the floor.

Bend your right knee and slowly move your pelvis forward until you feel a stretch in the calf and Achilles tendon of the left leg.

Hold for 15 seconds. Repeat with the other leg.

Warming Up

Stretching will help you warm up a bit, but it is most important to start your exercise very slowly. Don't start out at a jog or pumping the bike or stepper. Let the blood begin to flow gradually by getting started slowly and moving up steadily to your workout level.

The Size 2 Step-It-Up/Step-It-Down Program for Maximizing Caloric Burn

Start slowly. If you're doing the morning routine, then you'll probably still be half asleep and this shouldn't be a problem. Increase your pace in small increments (as explained later in the book) to a maximum comfortable exercise range and then decrease in regular intervals.

Finish off walking until your heart rate returns to normal. A pounding heart will force blood into the leg veins, and if the leg muscles are not pumping it back, the blood will collect there, potentially leading to vascular damage and varicose veins.

Sample Programs:

For illustration, here is an example for a person in good health, with no physical restrictions, looking to lose 20 lbs. and using the treadmill.

Step-It-Up

Start your warm up at 2.5 miles/hour for one minute. Increase to 3.0 miles/hour for two minutes, then increase to 3.5 miles/hour for two minutes. Next, increase your pace to jogging at 4.0 miles/hour for five minutes. Accelerate 0.5 miles/hour every five minutes, to a maximum speed that you can maintain comfortably for five minutes. *Do not overdue it!* Contrary to the "no pain, no gain" philosophies espoused by the popular, media hyped, 'fitness' shows, pushing yourself too far can put a quick end to your program through injuries as well as permanent damage to your joints, spine and cardiovascular system. Ignore these programs. They're not really concerned about your health - only improving their TV ratings.

Step-It-Down

This is a very important component, since here is where you'll greatly increase the total number of calories burned without stressing or straining yourself. From your maximum pace, decrease your speed 0.5 miles/hour for one to five minutes (depending on tolerance). Continue to decrease your pace 0.5 miles/hour every one to five minutes until you return to the 3.5 miles/hour pace, at which you'll be back to walking. Decrease your walking pace by 0.5 miles/hour every one to two minutes until you return to 2.5 miles/hour.

Continue this pace until your heart rate returns to near normal. Note the calories that you burned. By adding the Step-It-Down component, you will begin to burn an additional 10–30% more calories beyond what you would have burned on a typical Step-It-Up program alone. Over time, this will make a huge difference in how quickly you'll lose those extra pounds.

Motivation

Many people say they need a trainer to provide them with motivation. What they're really saying is that they're looking at their exercise program as a social alternative. Working with a trainer can be very social. At the rates they charge, they will be very conversant, understanding, and pleasant. Unfortunately, this won't help you get you to size 2 and truly help improve your social life. If you are planning on working with a trainer make sure that you still adhere to the 80/20 rule with most of your time spent doing calorie burning cardio. For example, if you've only got an hour per day to spend on exercise, spend 15 – 20 minutes with the trainer on strengthening and the rest on cardio – and preferably get the cardio in first. In fact, make sure that your trainer requires you to do so.

You can use the following methods to motivate you in your aerobic program. In addition, consider participating in some team sports or dancing programs, as mentioned later on.

Size 2 the TV – Turn on the Music

Let's face it: It's all about motivation. Television motivates you to sit around, not to exercise. It certainly won't motivate you to increase your pace during exercise. Nothing motivates like music with a beat. So turn off the TV and turn on the music. You'll see a dramatic increase in your motivation during exercise and will lose those extra pounds much faster.

Of course, there are exceptions. A friend of mine gets his motivation for cycling by watching the Playboy Channel. Hey, to each his own. Others get upbeat watching BET or other music video channels. Whatever works! But don't expect to get motivated by watching soaps or Talk Shows during your exercise. It's more likely that they'll keep your pace to a minimum.

The Beauty of Mirrors

Let your narcissistic qualities work for you. Don't hide in denial. Put a full-length mirror in front of your treadmill/stepper/bike/dance space. Accept what you look like now and plan what you're going to look like later. A touch of reality will go a long way to motivating you in your weight loss program. In the beginning and over time, the facts will speak for themselves and you'll slowly see the results as you witness the metamorphosis.

Dance, Dance, Dance

In front of the mirror by yourself, in a class, or out on the town. Better yet, all of the above. It's fun, social, and great exercise. It can also be invigorating, so make sure you're not overdoing the intensity. Remember, it's exercise and you need to follow the rules for aerobic exercise in general.

One caution: ADD IT TO YOUR AEROBIC PROGRAM, BUT DON'T USE IT AS A SUBSTITUTE until you can establish a regular routine. You can burn an additional 200–400 calories per dance session, or 600–800 calories per aerobics dance class – which, combined with your basic workout, will accelerate you to your goal. (See our Cardio Dance section later in the book for further insight and information.)

Weights/Resistance Training

Tone, don't bulk!

If your goal is to look like the Incredible Hulk then you're reading the wrong book. This program is designed for those who want to look lean and sexy, not buffed and intimidating.

My emphasis is to show you how to increase muscle tone and strength to support improved conditioning. Unless you plan to be a bodybuilder or furniture mover, forget the bulk. It won't help your health.

There's a lot of disagreement in the exercise community as to which is better: free weights, machines, or other weight-lifting methods. Again, from your standpoint it's all noise. Choose the resistance method you like best. Resistance bands, free weights, machines or simply using your own body weight will all get the job done.

For now, focus on working multiple muscle groups at light to moderate resistance, with more emphasis on repetitions. You should be able to comfortably do 10–15 repetitions without straining. Again, the key issue is not to injure yourself. Nothing will destroy your program quicker than injury.

For the novice weight lifter or newly activated former athlete, I prefer using the machines. Their responses are more controlled, and the risk of straining and injury should be lower.

There is also disagreement among the gurus as to how many sets should be done for each muscle groups, and which groups should be done in various orders and regimens. Whether you want to do two or three sets of certain machines or one set of every machine, the important point is that you do what you feel like doing on any particular day and not strain yourself doing so. I have to admit to some bias in doing one set of each of the different machines available. The logic is that you still get your exercise, but also tone a greater variety of muscles than you might otherwise. In any case, focus on the reps and put less emphasis on the weight.

For the initial prescription of resistance training, Dr. Williams and the researchers with the American Heart Association (AHA) recommend that "it should be performed in a rhythmic manner at a moderate to slow controlled speed. It should encompass a full range of motion. Breath-holding and straining (Valsalva maneuver) should be avoided by exhaling during the contraction or exertion phase of the lift and inhaling during the relaxation phase."

The researchers further state: "In addition, resistance training should alternate between upper and lower body work, allowing adequate rest between exercises. The initial weight load should not exceed 8 to 12 repetitions per set for healthy sedentary adults or 10 to 15 repetitions at a low level of resistance (e.g., less than 40% of 1-repetition maximum) for older individuals (aged > 50 to 60 years), more frail persons, or cardiac patients."

They further point out that: "At first, resistance training should not exceed a single set performed 2 days/week. It should involve the major muscle groups of the upper and lower extremities. Suitable exercises include chest press, shoulder press, triceps extension, biceps curl, pull-down (upper back), lower-back extension, abdominal crunch/curl-up, quadriceps extension or leg press, leg curls (hamstrings), and calf raise."

One last note: If you belong to a gym, make sure to ask a manager to provide you with information on how to use all of the equipment properly. Many people are shy to ask, but most gyms offer this service at no charge and some gyms provide "free" personal training sessions when you first join. Take advantage of this by bringing a notebook and writing down step-by-step instructions for each machine – just don't bother signing up for the extended training programs that they'll inevitably offer you.

Strength in Numbers?

Workout Buddies

Having someone to workout with seems like an obvious advantage. Unfortunately, relying on someone else to maintain your program can be inherently self-destructive. My advice is to build your program without any outside dependence or influence. If a buddy ends up coming along sometimes (or always), great – but don't make that person's participation a requisite to your program, or you risk turning their half-hearted motivation into excuses for breaking your own routine.

This is particularly important for the morning component. Let's face it, getting out of bed early every day is going to be hard enough to do yourself. Don't even think about expecting any other "fool" to join your "new religion." Keep the faith and save your own "soul" first. You can work on the rest of humanity later.

Even for the afternoon/evening component, my suggestion is that you have your buddy meet you at the gym (or other location), not go together. This way their excuses will not affect you. If they actually do show up, fine. My expectation is that 70% of the time they won't. Don't worry. Once they see how great you're looking, they'll follow.

Bottom line: Don't let your workout depend on anyone other than yourself. If you'd like to work out with your buddy, have your buddy join you. Or join a cardio class and make new buddies who are also dedicated to improving their health.

Don't have a treadmill? Can't or don't want to jog around the block? Want to alternate your exercise program each day? Please check out the new *Size 2 for Life – Total Fitness DVD*.

You can order via the web at: www.stancepublicatons.com

Real Results not Supercharged Fiction

Numerous studies have proven that in order to lose weight and keep it off a dieter needs to burn a minimum of 2000 – 2500 extra calories per week.   Despite this factual information a number of so-called "supercharged" programs have become popular by incorporating brief routines of interval training, totaling as little as 20 minutes or less per day. Based upon the magnitude of their book sales, to many dieters, the prospect of only a short period of exercise per day is apparently a very attractive proposition. Unfortunately, what these programs don't tell you is that a 20 minute interval workout is lucky to burn a mere 50 – 80 calories, very little of it from fat, but paradoxically leave you stiff with sore muscles.   Furthermore, although interval training can be a great adjunct to promote cardiovascular fitness it is not the best choice for the novice or re-starter, in my opinion. In *Size 2* we're committed to getting you where you want to go, not telling you what you want to hear. It's up to you to decide if you're happy with your present shape or really willing to make the commitment to becoming a frame adjusted size 2.

Fat calories are most efficiently burned in the training zone between 40 – 70% of maximal heart rate. Calories burned during the maximal heart rate zones of accelerated brief interval periods are mostly from the use of high energy phosphate molecules (ATP, PCr) that are held by the body in short supply. Once the body has consumed these it immediately draws on anaerobic glycolysis with the production of lactic acid. Very few calories are derived from fats during this process. Furthermore, during the cool down periods of interval training, the body turns to the next most readily available energy stores which are in the form of free glucose, lactate or glycogen. Again, very few fat calories are utilized.

The unique *Size 2* Step-It-Up/Step-It-Down program does the exact opposite. It focuses on maximal caloric burn from fat while also incorporating ample cardiovascular conditioning - without straining muscles and causing lactic acid production. In addition it does so at a pace that is easily tolerated by either the novice or the trained athlete, since the pace is adapted continuously according to an individual's own personal tolerance. Using the *Size 2* program you'll still spend sufficient time in the training range to promote cardiovascular conditioning but only as much as you can reasonably tolerate according to your current level of fitness. Over time though, you will quickly accelerate as your overall conditioning improves rapidly by avoiding the pains and strains that are so commonly a limiting factor, if not a primary reason for early termination of even the best intended weight lose aspirant. Add to this the fact that you'll be burning an additional 10 – 30% more fat calories during the easily tolerated Step-It-Down phase and you'll soon realize that the total fat calories burned will far surpass those of the so-called "supercharged" programs.

Please don't misunderstand. As mentioned above, interval training can be a great adjunct to a weight loss plan. We've even included a program of interval training that we feel addresses some of the above issues. But, if you think the popular 20 minute routines with their brief periods of rapidly accelerated intervals are sufficient to achieve or maintain weight loss, you may find yourself wholly disappointed.

Furthermore, starting out with interval training on your own is difficult and, in my opinion, not the best choice for the novice or re-starter. One primary reason is that it fails to take into consideration basic human nature. Let's face it; the first interval of an exercise session is hard enough to get motivated for at the outset, restarting after a cool down is downright near impossible. The practical fact is that most dieters will quit after the first interval cool down, only to have burned a mere 15 – 20 calories. On the other hand, appropriate level, group aerobic exercise classes, incorporating some interval training and conducted by trained instructors can be highly motivating and excellent routes to fitness if followed on a consistent basis.

Soon after you begin the *Size 2* Step-It-Up/Step-It-Down program you'll quickly realize that it addresses all the issues mentioned in this section from the outset. In the *Size 2* program you begin slowly and accelerate in easily tolerated stages – burning fat calories from the beginning. You also progress to a very tolerable cardiovascular conditioning phase while continuing to burn primarily fat calories. Then, in the Step-It-Down phase you maximize your session's caloric fat burn an additional 10 – 30% by progressively stepping down your pace in a manner that is easily tolerated even by the novice. The net effect: you maximize fat burn and improve cardiovascular conditioning without losing your motivation.

Now, enough supercharged nonsense, let's get started on the road to *Size 2*.

Getting Started

You should review the following program outlines and guidelines so that you have a general understanding of the program and where you fit in. Later on, we'll provide you with a day-by-day program that you can follow in detail. In the appendices, we'll also provide you with an easy-to-follow check sheet that you can copy and use during your journey to fitness.

Control Your Environment: At-Home Preparation

First, take a few minutes and eliminate temptation at home. Clear out all the junk food from your cupboards.

After you review the meal plan, stock up on the recommended ingredients to create healthy meals and snacks.

You've already taken the first step to fitness success. Each day, week, and month you'll build on this success to achieve your goals!

You should plan on a 30 - 40 minute morning exercise program and a 30 - 40 minute evening program. Over time, this should be increased to 40 - 60 minutes in the morning and 40 minutes or more in the evening, as your endurance and conditioning improves.

Evaluate Where You Stand

After assessing your overall health with your doctor, and taking into account any limitations he or she has advised you of, begin by assessing where you stand based on your weight.

What follows is a general outline of the program details based loosely on your fitness level and weight. Of course, you, in conjunction with your physician, should modify these according to your particular situation.

Group #1: I'm 5–20 pounds overweight

Morning:

Begin the first week with 10 minutes of walking, followed by 5 minutes of slow jogging and10 minutes of walking, then progress slowly and gradually from there.

Evening:

Begin with 10 minutes of walking on the treadmill, or 10 minutes on the bike or elliptical. Follow with 20 minutes of toning on the weight machines (or, at home, with resistance bands and/or free weights). Increase to walking and jogging or increase pace slowly over time.

After the first week, you can try a beginner aerobic dance or cardio class, with caution and without pushing yourself to keep up.

Group #2: I'm 20–40 pounds overweight

Morning:

Begin with 20 minutes of walking and five minutes of slow jogging, and progress very slowly from there. By the end of Phase 1 (Day 21), you should be able to increase your pace to that of Group #1.

Evening:

Begin with 10 minutes of walking on the treadmill, or 10 minutes on the bike or elliptical. Follow with 20 minutes of toning on the weight machines (or, at home, with resistance bands and/or free weights). Increase to walking and jogging or increase pace slowly over time.

Group #3: I'm 40–60 pounds overweight

Morning:

Begin walking 20–30 minutes and gradually increase your pace over the next 20 days. By Day 13, you may be able to walk for 15 minutes, jog for five minutes, and walk for five minutes more. By the end of Phase 1, you may be able to move on to Group #2.

Evening:

Begin with 10 minutes of walking on the treadmill, or 10 minutes on the bike or elliptical. Follow with 20 minutes of toning on the weight machines (or, at home, with resistance bands and/or free weights). Increase the pace slowly over time.

Group #4: I'm more than 60 pounds overweight

Morning:

Jogging should be avoided since it may cause damage to the spine, hips, and knees. It's best to combine walking and riding a stationary/semi-recumbent bicycle until ready to move on to Group #3. Start with walking for 20 minutes, and then a slow to moderate pace on the bicycle for 10 minutes.

Evening:

Begin with 10 minutes of walking on the treadmill, or 10 minutes on the bike or elliptical. Follow with 20 minutes of toning on the weight machines (or, at home, with resistance bands and/or free weights). Increase your walking pace slowly over time.

Remember: Consistency is the key to success!

Detailed Starting Exercise Program – Example

Aerobic (Morning) Program

This example will assume that you're using a home treadmill for your morning workout and that you're 20–40 pounds overweight. If you don't have a treadmill, going around the block repeatedly will suffice; just make sure you have running shoes with excellent cushioning. Alternatively, you can follow the program on the *Size 2 for Life – Total Fitness DVD*.

To adjust the program to your own circumstances just follow the above guidelines according to your group and adjust the intensity or increments in speed (.1 - .5) according to your own level of conditioning.

If you work, you'll need to get up a half hour to an hour earlier in the morning. What! Are you out of your mind? Sorry, yes, you heard me right – and yes, you'll curse me and yourself every morning. Just do it! When I was in practice, I had to be at work by 6:30 every morning. This meant getting up at 4:00 a.m. to workout. Boy was I p… But every day the scale went down and almost 60 pounds later nobody could even recognize me. I felt great!

If you're a "stay at home" parent or worker, then you don't need to get up earlier – but you do need to get you workout in before anything else (other than getting the kids off to wherever). Don't start anything. No phone calls. No housework. Nothing. If you do, then you'll never get to your workout, guaranteed. If you don't adhere to this simple principle, then your weight loss program could be doomed from the start.

Begin with some slow stretches, especially of the gastrocnemius muscle (back of your lower leg) and the Achilles tendon region. Don't bounce – just slow tension. Stretch and relax the muscles until they loosen up.

Get on the treadmill (or begin your walk outside) starting at a slow 2.5 miles per hour for one minute, and then increase the pace to 3.0 miles per hour for two minutes. You should be starting to wake up now, though still groaning a bit at yourself in the mirror. Increase the slope of the treadmill to a slight (.5) incline.

After two minutes, increase the pace to 3.5 miles per hour for another two minutes.

Now you can increase the pace to 4.0 miles per hour and do some very casual jogging for five minutes.

After five minutes, you'll increase your pace to 4.5 miles per hour for five more minutes. You may be tempted to increase your pace even more, now that you're awake and feeling good – but don't, at least not for the first week or two. Remember, injuries are your worst enemy and getting overly enthusiastic during the early phase will certainly lead to program-stopping injuries and pain. After the first two to three weeks, you can slowly and progressively increase your pace, but never to the point at which it leaves you in pain.

This is an important part. Make sure you do it every time you work out. It's called the Step–it-Down segment, and will result in your burning an extra 10–30% more calories – almost effortlessly. Drop the pace down to 4.0 miles per hour for another minute of slow jogging, and then after a minute down to 3.5 miles per hour for another minute more of brisk walking. Do the same the following minute by dropping the pace down to 3.0 miles per hour, and then in a minute down to 2.5. After a minute, you're done.

Good work! You're awake. You feel great and you're on your way. Not so bad, huh? Well, except for the waking up early part. Sorry, but you'll probably never really like that. Deal with it!

Note: At this point, if you're combining your initial morning/aerobic segment and your toning segment into a single integrated program then skip forward to the resistance section you've elected to follow (i.e. gym resistance component or resistance bands and stability ball). Alternatively, if you're pressed for time, check out our unique *Size 2 Express Core & Tone* section for amazingly fast results in just a few minutes per day.

Detailed (Evening) Resistance Program

Optional: Brief Warm-up Aerobic Component

This module will assume that you're in Group #2, including an evening workout in your program, and that you're working out at a local gym.

Arrive at the gym and begin with a five-minute warm up on either a bicycle or elliptical, if available.

Move over to a treadmill and make sure you again stretch out those calves, etc.

Begin the Step-It-Up component as in the morning exercise, and increase your pace in increments until you're jogging at 4.0–4.5 miles per hour for five-minute segments again.

Begin the Step-It-Down sequence and decrease your pace at the same rate as the morning program.

Congratulations! Adding even a brief additional aerobic component will greatly accelerate you toward your goal.

Note: If you're not following the morning aerobic program then you can easily add it in here by just extending the segment above to between 30 – 60 minutes depending upon your level of fitness and then going on to the following resistance segment.

Resistance Component

If you're new to resistance training, start with the lowest weight setting and add weight on gradually. Start out with 10 - 12 reps at a comfortable weight load. If you find that you can complete 12 reps easily, do 15 reps and remember to increase the weight a little next time to the point at which you can do 10 - 12 reps <u>without straining</u>.

Depending upon your available time, do 1-3 "circuits"[5] of the available machines. Each circuit should only take you between 10 - 15 minutes! Yes that's right; if you're pressed for time, you can be done with the resistance component in as little as 10 minutes and still have worked all the major muscle groups without bulking.

What follows is a simple example that should tone all the major muscle groups and give you an overall sense of balanced toning. You should be able to accomplish this at most gyms. Furthermore, most of the exercises work overlapping muscle groups, so, even if you only have time for one circuit, in effect you will still be doing multiple sets anyway.

Note: Every gym is laid out differently, so modify your routine to go conveniently from one machine to the next. Just try to work opposing or different muscle groups at each stop. For example, bicep curls followed by triceps presses or abdominal crunches, etc. Again, don't push it. The last thing you need is an injury.

One more thing: if you get to a machine and it's being used, just move on to the next exercise and come back to it later or on another day. There's plenty of overlap already built into the program. Just keep moving.

---

[5] One set of reps of each exercise.

Resistance Exercises

Shoulder Press
Targets: Deltoids, Triceps

Adjust seat so that handles are level with your shoulders.

Grasp handles and sit with your back against the pad.

Press handles overhead.

Return to start slowly.

Biceps Curl
Targets: Biceps

Adjust seat height so elbows align with the pivot point.

Grasp handles.

Keeping your arms on the pads, bend arms slowly and return with control.

Triceps Extension
Targets: Triceps

Adjust seat height so you can easily grasp the handles.

Keeping your back against the pad slowly push the handles forward/downward.

Return to start with control.

Deltoid Lift
Target: Deltoids and Trapezius Muscles

Chest Fly
Targets: Pectoralis Major, Anterior Deltoids

Adjust seat so that your elbows are slightly below your shoulders.

Grasp handles; push hands together while keeping forearms on the pad.

Chest Press
Targets: Pectorals, Anterior Deltoids. Triceps

Adjust height so handles are at the middle of your chest.

Free-weight Curls
At this point, I like to throw in a bit of light free-weight curls for 10–12 reps, since it's hard to find a really good curling machine.

Place hands on handles and press out, extending your arms fully while maintaining a slight bend in your elbows.

Return to start with control.

Angled Forward Press
Targets: Triceps, mid Deltoids and Pectorals

Rest back securely against back rest. Push forward slowly then slowly return to start.

Back Extension
Targets: Erector Spinae and Gluteus

Place feet under foot pad.

Extend back slowly and carefully without hyper extending.

 Return to start with slow control

Pull Down
Targets: Biceps. Latissimus Dorsi

Adjust eat to secure your legs under the pads.

Stand up and grasp handles

Sit down with legs under the pads.

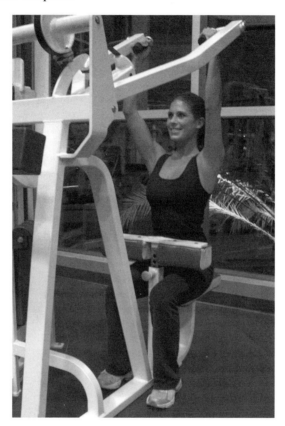

Pull handles down.

Straighten arms slowly as you return to the starting position.

Row Machine
Targets: posterior Deltoid, Trapezius, Rhomboids and Latissimus dorsi

Adjust seat to align chest with top of chest pad.

Sit tall with head and chest up and grasp the handles.

Pull the handles back slowly until elbows are by the hips.

Return with slow control.

Crunches

Finish off with a set of 10 - 30 crunches, as tolerated without straining.

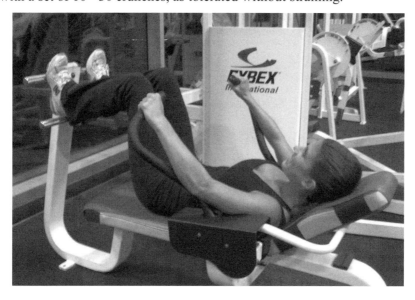

You're done!

You've just completed an overall toning of most of the major muscle groups. In time, you'll start to feel sleek and toned all over!

Wait! What about the legs?

I have to admit that here is where we perhaps cheat a bit – at least during the early phase of the program. It's not that we don't think that toning the legs is a good idea. It's just that 80% of the program already works the legs, and the notion that these exercises will localize the fat loss to the legs is false.

If you have time to add them, certainly do, but do so very cautiously and after the second or third week of the program. Overworking these areas can really tighten the muscles and make it very difficult to continue the aerobic component. Consider adding in these exercises on alternate days.

Ladies, if you want to really tone up those butts and thighs while reducing the appearance of cellulite then check out my stability ball exercise chapter. - Ashley

Leg Extensions
Target: Quadriceps Muscles

Hamstring Curls
Targets: Biceps Femoris; Gluteus

Gluteus Presses
Seated Leg Press

Targets: Quadriceps, Gluteus and Hamstrings

Adjust seat for desired range of motion.

Place feet on foot platform and lightly grasp the handles.

Slowly push against the foot platform until knees are slightly bent.

Return weight with a slow controlled movement.

Always keep knees lined up over toes.

Abductions/Adductions

If your gym has the following machine you can throw in some abductions and adductions for 10–12 reps.

Now Smile!

You've completed a full aerobic and resistance workout and have taken the first steps towards a lifelong *Size 2*.

No Gym Membership – No Problem

Do It Anywhere Cardio Exercises

This is a circuit-style workout, taking you through a series of cardio moves, with little or no rest between exercises. You can create more intensity by using a real jump rope or "imaginary" jump rope in between exercises instead of marching.

You will be doing each exercise for 2 minutes with a 30 second march/rope jump in-between.

- **Beginners**: You can substitute marching in place for any exercises that do not feel appropriate. Do not feel pressured to finish the 2-minute exercise and rest when you need to.
- **Intermediate**: Try to perform each exercise one after the other and alternate between marching and jump roping in-between exercises.
- **Advanced**: Jump rope in-between each exercise and repeat the entire routine.
- **Keep a water bottle nearby to ensure you stay hydrated.**
- **Optional Equipment**: Jump Rope and stable chair (with no wheels for the stretches)
- **Begin with some simple stretches.**

Hamstring Stretch

Extend one leg in front of you.

Keep both knees slightly bent.

Lengthen your torso as you bend over from the waist, lowering your upper body towards your extended leg.

Hold for 15 to 30 seconds and repeat on other leg.

*Option hold onto a chair for balance.

Quadriceps Stretch

Feet and legs hip width apart.

Place your right hand on the back of a chair for balance.

Grasp your left ankle or foot with your left hand.

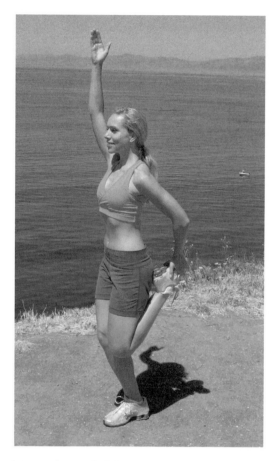

Gently pull your left heel toward your left buttock until you feel a stretch in the front of your thigh.

Hold 15 to 30 seconds and repeat on other leg.

*Option hold onto a chair for balance.

Calf Stretch

Stand with one foot in front of the other.

Bend the front leg while keeping the back leg straight.

Do not bounce.

Do not tense up.

Breathe deeply and let the calf loosen slowly.

Gently push your back heel to the floor.

Bend your forward knee until a comfortable stretch is felt in your back calf.

Hold for 15 to 30 seconds and repeat on other leg.

*Option hold onto a chair for balance.

Warm Up

Warm up by marching in place.

Bring the knees up to a comfortable level.

Don't overdo it by trying to bring the knees up too high too quickly.

Breathe in and out as you slowly accelerate your pace.

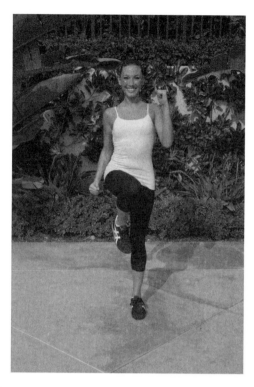

Keep marching and reach your arms overhead, alternating left and right.

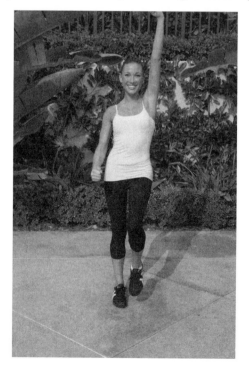

March wide, feet past the line of your hips.

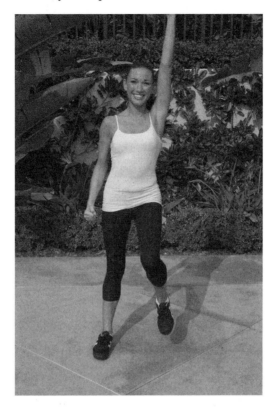

March wide, with alternating arms overhead.

Relax

Now relax, breathe deeply, in and out three times.

Now stretch. Bend your knees, reach up, and roll down to stretch your lower back. Round and contract your back four times. Repeat two times (1 minute).

Now, do each of the following drills for two minutes, then move on to the next.

Knees Up

March with knee raises

March right; raise your left knee toward your chest.

Alternate: March left, and raise your right knee to your chest.

After you feel comfortable with the knee raises, add intensity by reaching your arms up as you lift your knee and lower them as you march.

March or Jump Rope 30 seconds.

Sit Down

Imagine you are going to sit down on a chair. Lower your butt down into a squat position and stand up.

Once you feel confident doing the squat, add intensity by alternating knee raises as you stand up.

March or Jump Rope 30 seconds.

Walk It Up

March right, left tap, then march left, right tap.

To add intensity, lift the knee to the chest instead of tapping it on the floor. Take the march forward and back.

March or Jump Rope 30 seconds.

"Bionic Woman"

*One of my favorite butt exercises

Stand on your right foot; find your balance as you extend your left foot behind you.

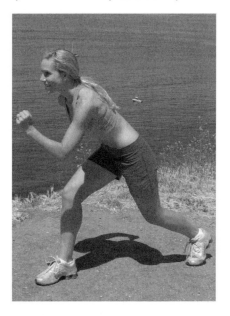

Keeping your right knee bent and your right knee over your right ankle tap your left toe to your right ankle.

Repeat for 30 seconds and switch legs.

Repeat 2 times on each leg.

March or Jump Rope for 30 seconds

"Box It"

Start in an upright position with the feet pointing straight, shoulder-width apart.

Make a fist with the hands and place them in front of your face.

Begin the movement by punching with the left hand to the right side.

Return to starting position

Repeat by punching the right hand to the left side.

Continue punching for 2 minutes.

March or Jump Rope 30 seconds

Skiers

This exercise simulates the motion of cross country skiing.

Start in an upright position with the legs in a staggered stance (one leg about 2 feet in front of the other).

One arm is raised opposite to leg (right leg forward, left arm raised).

Start the movement by switching the feet and the arms.

Repeat to the other side.

Keep alternating in a continuous fashion for 2 minutes.

March or Jump Rope 30 seconds

"Shuffles"

With your legs in a wide stance, shuffle your feet alternating right and left.

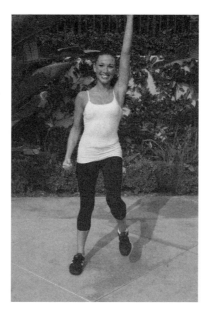

To add intensity, bring your arms up and down.

March or Jump Rope 30 seconds.

"Jack or Half Jack"

Do full jumping jacks.

Or alternate taps side to side while bringing arms overhead.

March or Jump Rope 30 seconds.

"Fancy Feet"

Alternate an imaginary jump rope, right, left double on the right.   Single, single, double switch left.

March or Jump Rope 30 seconds.

"Cancan Kicks"

Alternate kicks, keep them low and keep your abdominal muscles pulled in tight.

March or Jump Rope 30 seconds.

Cool Down

March in place (1 minute).

Continuing marching and rolling your shoulders to the back 8 times and forward 8 times. Slow your march down for 1 minute.

March wide and alternate toe taps right and left.

Keep your legs wide and inhale reaching the arms overhead.

Exhale as you bring your arms down

Repeat 4 times.

Relax, take several deep breaths and then repeat the initial stretch routine.

At Home Resistance Training

You can get an excellent resistance-training workout at home, with or without any equipment. I guarantee everyone has at least one piece of resistance equipment already – YOU! Your own body weight provides excellent resistance. Think of a push-up; many top trainers regard this as a near-perfect exercise. Take a look around – what other things are already in your house, like stairs, a chair, or water jugs? Be creative. I often train clients at their homes, and some of them do have beautifully equipped home gyms, but I also train people with nothing but the little bag of tricks I bring with me – a stability ball and a set of resistance bands. Guess what? The fancy equipment doesn't make the difference – it is the energy, form, and focus you put into it.

There are tons of options if you want to create an at-home gym, and if you have the money, I say go for it. I see many benefits of training at home:

Nobody cares what you look like (you can work out in your pj's).

No wasted time driving to and from the gym.

No waiting in line to use sweaty equipment.

No excuses that the gym is closed – if you're up at 3 a.m., you can do it then.

But before you go out and spend a lot of money on fancy gym equipment, you may want to start slowly and make sure you really need it. I'd hate to have you using that $1,500 Bowflex as a clothes hanger.

For less than $50, you can get two of my favorite training tools: a resistance band and a stability ball. That's less than a month's membership at many health clubs. Most of the resistance band sets and stability balls even come with workout posters, and some include an instructional DVD.

Why Resistance Bands?

Bands are great because they are cheap, compact, portable and versatile.

Because resistance bands are so compact and lightweight, you can easily take them along when you travel or if you want to sneak in a mini "at workout." Resistance bands generally come in three or four different levels of resistance and cost about $15 per band.

Yellow (thin)

Red (medium)

Green (heavy)

Blue (extra heavy)

Resistance Band Exercises

Beginners 2 sets of 12 repetitions of each exercise

Intermediate- 3 sets of 12 repetitions

Advanced- 3 sets of 15 repetitions

Remember you need to warm up first with 5-10 minutes of light aerobic exercise and stretch after.

Breathing: People tend to hold their breath when they are doing resistance exercise, which can be dangerous. Breathing is very important during exercise.

Exhale fully on the exertion phase of the lift. The exertion phase is the hardest part.

Inhale deeply on the easier phase, the release or the return to the starting position.

Resistance Band Squats

Great exercise to get ready for ski season! – Dr. Mel Reich, Episode Host, Lifetime TV

Start by stepping on the resistance band with both feet.

Try to use a shoulder width stance if you can. - Ashley

Hold the resistance band at shoulder level with both hands.

Start into a full squat while holding the band at shoulder height.

Return to the starting position and repeat.

Chest Press

Wrap the band around a sturdy object behind you at chest level.

Secure band around a pole, tree or post. Stand with back to tree, feet slightly more than shoulder-width apart Holding the handles of the bands, extend both arms forward.

Holding handles of band, extend both arms forward.

Then alternate chest press

Keep the right arm stationary and press the left arm out.

Bring the left arm back and then press forward with the right arm.

Lat Pull

Stand with feet shoulder-width apart, holding a band securely underneath the feet.

Hold one end of band in each hand.

Lean forward at the waist so torso is parallel to the floor, arms bent 90 degrees.

Contract the back and pull the band out while bringing the elbows towards the sky.

Return to start position.

Biceps Curls with Resistance Band

Stand with feet shoulder width apart, knees slightly bent, and at a staggered stance.

Step onto middle of tubing with back foot or both feet. Grasp ends with underhand grip with arms hanging down at sides. Elbows should be close to sides.

Flex at the elbows and curl band up to approximately shoulder level. Keep elbows close to sides throughout movement.

Return to start position.

Pull Over's with Resistance Band

Secure band around a pole, tree or post. Start by holding the handles in both hands. Lean forward at waist, keeping back straight. Pull the band towards your hips, as if you were paddling on a surf board.

Extend from your elbow until your arm is fully extended.

Return to the start position.

Resistance Band Single Arm Rows

Start by placing the band under one foot and stepping backwards with the other foot. Bend over keeping your back flat at a 45-degree angle.

Pull the bands up towards your waist keeping your elbows in close together.

Squeeze your shoulder blades together when performing rowing motion.

Return to start position.

Standing Rows with Resistance Band

Secure band around a sturdy object.

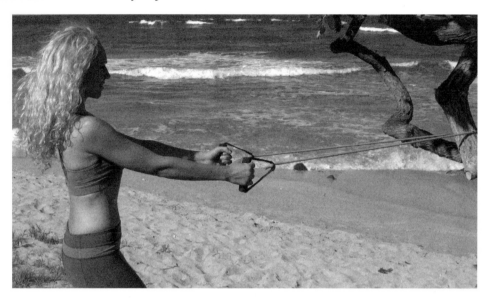

Secure band around a pole, tree or post. Start position: Grasp ends with a neutral grip (palms facing each other).

Raise band to side of body at shoulder height keeping elbows slightly bent.

Slowly pull the bands to your hips. Return to start.

Torso Twist

Secure band around a pole, tree or post. Turn your upper body away from the object by twisting, without moving the legs.

Return to starting position. Repeat on opposite side.

Stability Ball

(Swiss, Balance, Stretch, and Physio Ball)

I don't care what you call it, just as long as you use it! If you want to purchase only one affordable piece of equipment, get a stability ball. It can provide a great upper-body workout, a lower-body workout, a challenging abdominal workout, and can assist your stretching. How many things improve your balance and posture merely by sitting on them? Because the stability ball is an unstable surface, you have to use all of your stability muscles in your core just to balance.

If you already have dumbbells, you can also use the stability ball as a weight bench.

Beginners – two sets of 12 repetitions of each exercise

Intermediate – three sets of 12 repetitions of each exercise

Advanced – three sets of 15 repetitions of each exercise

Remember, you need to warm up first with 5–10 minutes of light aerobic exercise, and stretch after.

General recommended size-to-height for stability ball selection is as follows:

55 cm. ball	21 inches	4' 11" - 5' 4" tall
65 cm. ball	25 inches	5' 5" to 5' 11" tall

Stability Ball Exercises

Sitting on the Stability Ball

First, sit comfortably on the ball. You may want to begin with a wall or stable counter nearby, in case you lose your balance. Your feet should be wide on the floor; this makes it easier to balance. Contract your abdominals by pulling your belly button toward your spine, and begin moving your hips slightly side to side, then in small circles – in one direction, and then the other.

Ball Push-Ups

Roll forward, placing your body weight on your hands until stability ball rests under your shins. Your body should be extended in a straight line from the stability ball.

Lower your upper body toward floor, bending at the elbows to perform push-ups. Keep the abdominal muscles tight. Keep the body tight and straight from shoulders to toes.

Return to start position. To increase difficulty, roll the ball back so only your feet are resting on it.

Abdominal Crunches

Lie with the ball resting under the mid-lower back and place hands behind the head or across the chest.

Contract your abs to lift your torso off the ball, pulling the bottom of your rib cage down toward your hips.

As you curl up, keep the ball stable. Return to start.

Inner Thighs and Abdominals

Lie on your side with the ball between your knees or ankles, squeezing it to hold it in place.

Squeeze your inner thighs and contract the waist and hip muscles to lift the ball in the air.

Lie on your back with the ball between your knees or ankles, squeezing it to hold it in place. Keep your hips stacked and abs tight to stabilize your body.

Squeeze your inner thighs and contract the waist and hip muscles to lift the ball in the air.

Return to start.

Back Extension

Position the ball under your hips and lower torso, with your knees straight or bent. Slowly roll down the ball.

Lift your chest off the ball, bringing your shoulders up until your body is in a straight line. Make sure your body is in alignment (i.e., head, neck, shoulders, and back are in a straight line), your abs are pulled in, and you don't hyperextend the back.

Return to start.

Butt Raises

Lie on the ball with the head, neck, and shoulders supported, knees bent, and body in a "tabletop position" across the ball.

Lower the hips toward the floor without rolling on the ball.

Squeeze the glutes to raise hips until body is in a straight line, like a bridge.

Hold weights on the hips for added intensity, and make sure you press through the heels and not the toes.

Good Job!

Size 2 Express Core & Tone

Think you don't have time to exercise today or need to keep things brief? If you have 10 minutes (I know you do) the *Size 2 Express Core & Tone* program is just for you. Get an overall body-toning and core workout in less than 10 minutes.

All you'll need are two light hand weights, a comfortable rug or mat and as little as 10 minutes of time.

Notes:

- To maximize results the sequences below should be completed in a smooth, progressive fashion - one step flowing into the next.
- Choose weights that allow you to do 12 biceps curls with only <u>slight</u> straining on your 12th repetition.
- Exhale when you contract your muscles and inhale when you relax. For example: exhale as you raise your arms during a biceps curl and inhale as you lower your arms.
- Also note that you will be using different muscle groups for sequential exercises so you should need little or no rest in between.

Standing Sequence

Biceps Curls (front of upper arms)
Start with elbows by your side and arms extended. Slowly curl both arms at the same time. Return to start. Repeat 10 times.

Overhead Arm Presses (shoulders and arms)

Bend both arms with weights held at shoulder lever. Slowly extend both arms at the same time above your head. Return to start. Repeat 10 times.

Biceps Hammer Curls (front of upper arms)

Bring your arms back down along your sides, palms facing towards your body. Raise your arms until your forearms are parallel with the floor. Slowly lower your arms to the starting position. Repeat 10 times.

Weighted Squats (front of your legs)

Now with your arms and weights still by your side, stand with your feet hip width apart. Shift your hips backwards and lower yourself until your thighs are parallel (or almost parallel) to the floor. Make sure you keep your abdominals contracted. Push through your feet with the weight in your heels back up to standing. Repeat 10 times.

Overhead Press/Triceps Extensions (back of upper arms)

With one weight held by both hands behind your head at neck level, press the dumbbell overhead, extending your elbows until your arms are vertical to the floor, elbows pointing forward. Slowly lower the dumbbell behind your head to the starting position. Repeat 10 times.

Weighted Plies (inner thighs)

Continuing with one weight held by both hands. Step out into a wide stance with toes turned out. Bend your knees to a 90-degree (or almost 90 degree angle). Squeeze your butt to stand back up. Repeat 10 times.

Mat Sequence

Mat Crunches (abdominals)

Lie on you back with your feet on the floor and your knees bent upward about 60 degrees. Contract your abdominal muscles to lift your shoulders off the mat. Return to start. Repeat 10 - 30 times.

*Option: place your hands behind your head for neck support.

Butt Lifts (butt, back of legs and lower back)
Stay on your back with your knees bent and your heels on the floor.

Raise your buttocks off the floor until your back forms a straight line from knees to shoulders, and hold for 1 second before lowering to the starting position. Repeat 10 times.

Lying Leg lifts (abdominals)
Extend your legs on the matt. Slowly raise your legs six inches - one foot off the floor.

Hold this position for ten seconds. Return to start. Repeat 10 times.

Leg side lifts (outer thigh, hip muscles, abdominals)
Roll onto your side with your bottom arm extended below and above your head. Your hips should be stacked, legs long with a slight bend in the knee.

Raise the upper leg away from the lower leg with control, keeping your abdominals pulled in. Return to start. Repeat 10 times.

Roll over and repeat the sequence for the opposite side.

Back Extension (abdominals and lower back)
Roll on to your stomach. Pull your abdominals in and keep them contracted throughout the exercise.

Extend your arms and squeeze your back to lift your chest and legs a few inches off the floor. Hold this position 3 – 10 seconds.

Return to start. Repeat 10 times.

Lower back stretch

With your shins on the floor slowly rest your chest on the knees. Stretch your arms forward and allow your forehead to rest on your mat. Let you back relax and inhale several times. Maintain this position for 20 – 30 seconds.

Plank (abdominals, back and chest)

Lie face down on your mat resting on the forearms; make a fist with your hands.

Push off the floor, raising up onto toes and resting on the elbows. Maintain a straight line from head to heels. Contract your abdominals; imagine trying to pull your navel to the ceiling.

Hold for10 - 60 seconds.

Push-ups (arms, shoulders and chest)

Starting Position: Kneel on an exercise mat or floor and bring your feet together behind you.

Place your palms flat on the mat, positioning your hands shoulder-width apart, shoulders directly over your hands.

Lower your body towards the mat until your chest or chin touches the mat. Press upwards until your arms are fully extended at the elbows. Return to start. Repeat 10 – 20 times.

Repeat lower back stretch.

Congratulations!

You just did a complete core strengthening and toning program in less than 10 minutes.

Have a bit more time?

Repeat either or both sequences now or whenever you have a little bit of free time for even faster results. As you can see, it's quick and easy!

Putting It All Together

The 21-Day Size <u>2</u> for Life Diet & Fitness Program

Get Ready to Change How You Look and Feel in Just 21 Days

The 21-Day Size 2 for Life Diet & Fitness Program is the time to challenge yourself and create a new you. This is the most restrictive part of the program. You will be following this meal and exercise plan for 21 days. This is the time to break unwanted "food addictions" and retrain your body and mind to crave healthy foods.

*Warning: This intensive program is not advisable for anyone suffering from a medical condition, or for pregnant or lactating women. Seek the advice of your doctor before beginning any diet program.

Why 21 Days?

Because 21 days of dedicated thought and consistent action, toward the change you want, will create a desired habit while replacing an unwanted behavior.

Dr. Maxwell Maltz (1899–1976) wrote the bestseller *Psycho-Cybernetics*. Originally a plastic surgeon, Maltz noticed that it took 21 days for amputees to cease feeling phantom sensations in the amputated limb. From further observations, he found it took 21 days to create a new habit.

Brain circuits take engrams (memory traces), and produce neuro-connections and neuro-pathways only if they are bombarded for 21 days in a row. This means that our brain does not accept "new" data for a change of habit unless it is repeated each day for 21 days, without missing a day.

The new habit needs to take the place of a previously entrenched old one. Old habits are not so easily overruled. The new habit will need to be supported and encouraged to have any chance of survival.

21-Day Transformation Steps

Make the decision.

See It

Create the image of your goal in your mind. Take a few minutes each day to visualize your goal. See yourself overflowing with health and energy. You may want to use a picture of yourself at your ideal weight, a picture from a magazine, the number you want to see on the scale, or the clothing size you want to wear.

Say It

Choose the habit you most want to focus on for the next 21 days. Repeat an auto-suggestion phrase 20 times when you wake up and 20 times before you go to sleep.

Example: Habit – Eating late at night.

"I only eat before seven p.m.; I am in control of when I eat; I no longer eat after seven p.m."

Write It

Writing down your goal is a commitment to achieve it. Taking the time to focus, visualize, and write down your specific goal creates momentum that will fuel your actions. Write your goal as if it has already been achieved: I am so happy now that _____.

Success Strategies

In order for you to maximize your weight loss and fitness program, it's highly recommended that you follow these suggestions:

Exercise: This program should be integrated with The 21-Day Size 2 for Life Fitness Program.

Water: Please remember to drink 8–10 glasses of filtered water each day.

Alcohol: If at all possible, avoid alcohol. Cutting out alcohol, especially during the first 21 days, can add an additional two to three pounds of weight loss per week and greatly increase your energy level.

Stop Eating At Least Three Hours Before Going To Sleep: By imposing an eating cut-off time of three (or more) hours before bed, we automatically slash our caloric intake, commonly cutting 500–1000 calories per day, which can add up to an additional two pounds of additional weight loss per month.

Combine these two, and you'll be looking at an additional five pounds of weight loss per week.

The best way to get rid of an unwanted habit is to replace it with a good habit for 21 consecutive days.

Food List

Make sure to stock up on the following items:

Vegetables: Asparagus, Bell Pepper, Bok Choy, Broccoli, Brussels Sprouts, Cabbage, Cauliflower, Celery, Chard, Collard Greens, Cucumber, Eggplant, Kale, Mushrooms, Onion, Peppers, Radishes, Spinach, Sprouts, String Beans, Yellow Squash, Zucchini

Note: A number of fast and simple microwavable vegetable combinations have come available lately. Stock up and use them for the vegetable portion of your meals. Also feel free to substitute them as a great alternative snack any time of the day. – Dr. Paulsen

Lettuce: Romaine, endive and similar leafy greens, iceberg

Toppings/Mixers: Mustard, salsa, low-calorie flavored/unflavored water for mixing your smoothies, nonfat whey or soy protein powder. Also, pick up some whole psyllium husk to sprinkle into your sauces, mixes and smoothies. The added fiber has many health benefits in addition to providing an easy way to reduce your appetite while improving your gastrointestinal function.

Meats: Chicken breast, fish, turkey, lean steak, lean lamb, pork tenderloin, extra-lean turkey slices, extra-lean chicken slices, and eggs

Meat Substitutes: BOCA burgers or other soy burgers with less than four grams of fat per serving, tofu, tempeh, low-fat soy cheese, low-fat soy yogurt, eggs, soybeans

Fruits: Blueberries, Strawberries, Blackberries, Boysenberries, Raspberries, Apples, Pears, Nectarines, Melon, Oranges, Peaches, Grapefruit, Kiwi, Plums, Tangerines

Notes: During the first 7–21 days, any between-meal snacks should preferably be boiled egg whites or 99% fat-free turkey breast, ham, or chicken slices and topped with mustard, if desired. Fruit can be eaten sparingly during the first 7–21 days, after which it can be added more liberally.

Although the meal plans contain sufficient nutrients, adding in a multi-vitamin supplement is acceptable, but, stay clear of the mega-dose formulas.

Snack Options

Each snack should be between 170–200 calories:

> Popcorn (oil-free and unsalted) cooked in a no-oil microwave bowl popper (Note: you can pick one up at Target) or air popper. *Not prepackaged microwave popcorn!*
> Uncooked (soft) whole wheat or multi grain tortillas to be toasted in a toaster oven
> 1 serving fruit
> 1 serving string cheese with small fruit
> 1 oz. roast turkey wrapped round celery or carrot sticks
> 3 oz. fresh tuna with 2 cups of lettuce
> 1 cup veggies with 2 Tbsp. nonfat dressing
> 2 cups salad with 2 Tbsp. nonfat dressing
> Whey protein shake
> 1/2 cup nonfat cottage cheese with small fruit
> Hardboiled egg whites

General Notes

If you do the aerobic exercise program in the morning as recommended, you may not be hungry for a fair part of the morning. If you're at the office or out on the road, you'll likely have a mid-morning meal instead of breakfast. Plan for this with a selection of pre-prepared protein smoothies.

Preparing for the 21-Day *Size 2 for Life* Diet & Fitness Program

Strategic Plan

"People with goals succeed because they know where they are going." – Earl Nightingale

During the next 21 days, you'll transform your old behaviors/habits and create new ones to support your goals. Each day, for 21 consecutive days, you will be using the 21-Day Size 2 for Life Program to establish your new healthy lifestyle goals.

The first step in making a real commitment is your belief in yourself; "I am doing this," instead of "I'm going to try to do it." The language you use is just as important as your physical action. Create an inner and outer dialogue that is focused on the results you want. Know that you have the power to change your behavior and create the outcome you desire.

Take a few minutes to answer the following questions, writing down the first three answers that come to mind:

Why do you want to change your body?

1.

2.

3.

What is preventing you from achieving your goal?

1.

2.

3.

You Can Do It!

Start with a Personal Success Contract. Read the following contract, which you'll be making with yourself and resolve to honor it from now on. Energize your goal today by signing your contract.

Personal Success Contract

I, _____ , commit to starting my fitness program today, _____.

I commit to using the Size 2 for Life – Change Your Life Workout Program consistently and following the *Size 2 for Life* healthful eating program that will help me attain my fitness and health goals.

I will only fuel my body with the most nutritious foods possible.

I will be kind to myself and appreciate all that my body does for me.

I will strive to challenge my body and my mind.

I will acknowledge and reward myself for my achievements along the way.

_____

Signature

Day One

"A goal is nothing more than a dream with a deadline."

Action Step

Energize your goal today by signing your Success Contract and beginning The 21-Day Size 2 for Life Diet & Fitness Plan.

Morning weigh in (It all begins here!)

Morning exercise

Breakfast or Mid-morning Meal

Coffee/tea/personal choice

Blended smoothie with 1–2 scoops protein powder

OR:

6–10 hardboiled egg whites

6 oz. vegetable juice

Lunch

One 6-8 oz grilled skinless chicken breast

Steamed broccoli and cauliflower

Iced tea/natural low calorie soda

Afternoon Snack

Protein smoothie

Evening exercise

Aerobics dance class/elliptical trainer/treadmill/bike; plus 20 minutes of toning

Evening weigh in

Dinner

6-8 oz grilled salmon

Steamed vegetables

Sparkling mineral water/iced tea/water

Evening Snack – optional

Unsalted microwave oil-free popcorn

Raw vegetables (celery sticks, baby carrots, broccoli, etc.) with fat-free dressing dip, if desired

Day Two

"You must first see a thing in your mind before you can do it." – Alex Morison

Action Step

Take a few minutes today and visualize the body you want. Create the image in rich detail, focusing on the positive changes that are occurring now. You may want to use real pictures, as well – a favorite prior photo of yourself, a body you admire that will remind you of your goal.

Take action by eating a healthy breakfast. People who regularly skip breakfast are four times as likely to be obese than those who eat breakfast. Breakfast eaters consume less fat during the day and have lower cholesterol levels than those who don't.

NOTE: If you follow the Size 2 for Life morning exercise program and don't feel hungry for a while afterward, prepare for this with a pre-made mid-morning breakfast or nutritious smoothie. Don't wait until lunch to eat – your resistance to "pigging out" will be insurmountable.

Morning weigh in

Morning exercise

Breakfast or Mid-morning Meal

Coffee/tea/or personal choice

Blended smoothie with 1–2 scoops protein powder

OR:

Egg white omelet with salsa

6 oz. vegetable juice

Lunch

6-8 oz roasted skinless turkey breast

Mixed salad with fat-free dressing, if needed or steamed vegetables

Iced tea/natural low calorie soda

Afternoon Snack

Protein smoothie

Evening exercise

Aerobics dance class/elliptical trainer/treadmill/bike; plus 20 minutes of toning

Evening weigh in

Dinner

6-8 oz grilled halibut

Steamed vegetables

Sparkling mineral water/iced tea/water

Evening Snack – optional

Baked/toasted tortilla and salsa

Cherry tomatoes and cucumber slices with fat-free dressing dip, if desired

Day Three

Action Step

Decide what you want. Decide what you are willing to exchange for it.

Step One

Each day, take a look at one behavior you want to change.

Step Two

Write a list of the reasons why you want to change.

Step Three

Write one action you will take NOW to change that behavior and how you will feel when you are free from the behavior.

EXAMPLE

Step One

Quit snacking when I watch TV.

Step Two

Eating mindlessly makes me feel bad – I could be doing other things – I don't feel productive – it wastes my time.

Step Three

I will not eat when I watch TV.

I feel proud of myself!

The average American spends 30–40 hours per week watching TV – a completely sedentary activity. If you are watching TV, make commercial breaks a mini workout – stretch, march in place, do a quick set of squats, or even jumping jacks.

Morning weigh in

Morning exercise

Breakfast or Mid-morning Meal

Coffee/tea/or personal choice

Blended smoothie with 1–2 scoops protein powder

OR:

Scrambled egg whites with peppers and onions

6 oz. vegetable juice

Lunch

6-8 oz lean steak

Steamed broccoli and cauliflower

Iced tea/natural low calorie soda

Afternoon Snack

Protein smoothie

Evening exercise

Aerobics dance class/elliptical trainer/treadmill/bike; plus 20 minutes of toning

Evening weigh in

Dinner

6-8 oz grilled haddock

Steamed cauliflower

Sparkling mineral water/iced tea/water

Evening Snack – optional

Four extra lean ham slices topped with mustard.

Raw vegetables (celery sticks, baby carrots, broccoli, etc.) with fat-free dressing dip, if desired

Day Four

"Your focus is everything." – William James

Action Step

Today, focus on all the positive actions you are taking to attain your healthy ideal body.

Step One

Close your eyes and create a feeling of certainty that you will achieve your goal.

Step Two

Take a deep breath. As you exhale, release any doubt, fear, or limiting beliefs that may have blocked you from reaching your goal in the past.

Step Three

Open your eyes with a feeling of certainty that your goal will be achieved.

Repeat this process each morning and evening.

Morning weigh in

Morning exercise

Breakfast or Mid-morning Meal

Coffee/tea/or personal choice

Blended smoothie with 1–2 scoops protein powder

OR:

Egg white cheese omelet with fat-free cheese and tomatoes

6 oz. vegetable juice

Lunch

4 oz lean hamburger with mustard, lettuce, tomato, and onion, without the bun

Iced tea/natural low calorie soda

Afternoon Snack

Protein smoothie

Evening exercise

Aerobics dance class/elliptical trainer/treadmill/bike; plus 20 minutes of toning

Evening weigh in

Dinner

6-8 oz baked skinless chicken breast

Steamed vegetables

Sparkling mineral water/iced tea/water

Evening Snack – optional

Baked/toasted tortilla and salsa

Day Five

"We are what we think about all day long." – Ralph Waldo Emerson

Your thoughts are in your control, and they can be very powerful. Positive thoughts can motivate healthy behaviors, such as eating right and being active. It's simple, really. If you believe you can take 10,000 steps a day, you will be more likely to take an extra walk to meet your goal.

But the reverse is also true. Your thoughts can be defeating. "I've already messed up on my meal plan, so it doesn't matter if I eat a second piece of cake."

Negative thoughts and negative self-talk may sabotage your good intentions. Positive thinking can help you achieve and maintain healthy behaviors.

Studies have measured the success of positive thinkers and found that those who think they can lose weight, or increase their physical activity, do! These people are more successful than people with less faith in themselves. The confidence you have in performing a certain behavior is called self-efficacy, and self-efficacy is a key in successful behavior change.

Action Step

Want Results?

Can-Do!

Many professional athletes get top sports training and coaching in positive thinking to help them achieve their goals. And it works! The same can apply for you and me. A "can-do" attitude may be just what it takes to jumpstart a healthier lifestyle. Best of all, your attitude is something you can control.

You have the choice to have a positive outlook. Chances are, when you choose to think positively, you'll feel better about yourself and be able to perform better in whatever you do.

Stay On Track

There will be days when you don't feel like working out, slip from eating right, or lose your temper. Small setbacks are part of life. Learn from your past successes and failures.

Don't dwell on the past. Learn and move on, so next time you'll make healthier choices toward positive change.

How to Stay Positive

Positive thinkers admit when they feel frustrated or depressed. They don't ignore it. But they also don't blame themselves. Instead, they try to understand the negative thoughts and feelings, and counter them with more positive ones.

So, how do you stay positive, maintain momentum, and sustain healthy behaviors?

1. Take a minute to give yourself an ego boost. Repeat some motivational words out loud or to yourself.

2. Avoid negative talk, such as "I'm not good at this." It's dangerous for your well-being and healthy goals. Try to avoid the negative inner voice.

3. Remind yourself that you deserve happiness and are making positive changes.

Get support. Tell your friends and family about your healthy habits. It helps to have a supportive network. But remember, don't become reliant on anyone else to achieve your goals.

Reward yourself. Give yourself a pat on the back for all your healthy efforts. Get a massage, go to a show, or enjoy a new DVD or CD.

Have a plan. Making a plan to exercise or eat healthy lunches can mean the difference between sticking with your goals or falling off track. If you've planned for an activity, you are likely to stick with it. Take it day by day or week by week.

The process of writing down your personal action plan is a good way to keep you honest, watch your progress, or notice your pitfalls.

Think positive thoughts while you work out. Use thoughts like "The world looks good. I'm glad I'm training today. I feel great." Avoid thoughts like "I'm tired. I'm not improving." Remember that your training session is probably the only time you'll have all day that's just for you. You want it to be as pleasant, positive, and productive as possible.

Morning weigh in

Morning exercise

Breakfast or Mid-morning Meal

Coffee/tea/or personal choice

Blended smoothie with 1–2 scoops protein powder

OR:

6–10 hardboiled egg whites

6 oz. vegetable juice

Lunch

Two-cheese (fat-free) skinless chicken breast tacos with salsa

Iced tea/natural low calorie soda

Afternoon Snack

Protein smoothie

Evening exercise

Aerobics dance class/elliptical trainer/treadmill/bike; plus 20 minutes of toning

Evening weigh in

Dinner

6-8 oz skinless Cornish hen

Mixed salad with fat-free dressing, if needed

Sparkling mineral water/tea/water

Evening Snack – optional

Unsalted microwave oil-free popcorn

Cherry tomatoes and cucumber slices with fat-free dressing dip, if desired

Day Six

"Every day I count wasted in which there has been no dancing." – Friederich Nietzsche

Action Step

Fitness has many forms. Add a physical activity that you enjoy – hiking, biking, dancing, swimming, yoga, or a walk in a beautiful setting. Fully immerse yourself in it and feel the rhythm of it. Look for new opportunities to move more every day. Our bodies are gifts. The fitter we become, the more we can fully experience the joy of movement each day.

Morning weigh in

Morning exercise

Breakfast or Mid-morning Meal

Coffee/tea/or personal choice

Blended smoothie with 1–2 scoops protein powder

OR:

6–10 hardboiled egg whites

6 oz. vegetable juice

Lunch

6-8 oz grilled skinless chicken breast

Steamed green beans and carrots

Iced tea/natural low calorie soda

Afternoon Snack

Protein smoothie

Evening exercise

Aerobics dance class/elliptical trainer/treadmill/bike; plus 20 minutes of toning

Evening weigh in

Dinner

Broiled cod

Steamed vegetables

Sparkling mineral water/iced tea/water

Evening Snack – optional

Baked/toasted tortilla and salsa

Day Seven

"Discipline means choices. Every time you say yes to a goal or objective you say no to many more." – Sybil Stanton

Action Step

You can always make a healthy choice.

Commit to make the best health choices possible – even at the drive-through window.

Morning weigh in

Morning exercise

Breakfast or Mid-morning Meal

Coffee/tea/or personal choice

Blended smoothie with 1–2 scoops protein powder

OR:

2 low-fat soft tacos with 4 (2+2) hardboiled eggs whites with fat-free cheese and salsa. Microwave taco sized tostadas and cheese then add chopped egg whites and warm salsa.

6 oz. vegetable juice

Lunch

Two 6-8 oz grilled skinless chicken breasts

Iced tea/natural low calorie soda

Afternoon Snack

Protein smoothie

Evening exercise

Aerobics dance class/elliptical trainer/treadmill/bike; plus 20 minutes of toning

Evening weigh in

Dinner

6 oz grilled lean ham steak

Mixed salad with fat-free dressing, if needed

Sparkling mineral water/tea/water

Evening Snack – optional

Four rolled turkey slices with/without mustard

Raw vegetables (celery sticks, baby carrots, broccoli, etc.) with fat-free dressing dip, if desired

Day Eight

"Success is the sum of small efforts, repeated day in and day out."– Robert Collier

Action Step

Get moving! Everything counts when it comes to physical activity.

Sixty minutes of "The Size 2 for Life" workout will burn between 400–700 calories.

Walking – 10 minutes of brisk walking will burn approximately 100 calories.

Swimming – 10 minutes of swimming laps will burn 100 calories.

Biking – 20 minutes will burn 100 calories.

Stairs – climbing stairs for 20 minutes will burn approximately 100 calories.

Housework – 20 minutes will burn approximately 100 calories.

Gardening – 20 minutes will burn approximately 100 calories.

All of these "small efforts" can really make a difference at the end of the month. If you add one per day, along with three Size 2 for Life aerobic sessions, that's approximately 4,200 calories burned per month.

Check out http://www.healthstatus.com to find out how many calories you burn doing other activities.

Morning weigh in

Morning exercise

Breakfast or mid-morning meal.

Whey protein shake mixed with 5 oz. nonfat milk, soy milk, or half milk and half water; mix in a blender with ice.

OR:

Egg white omelet

> 6 egg whites, lightly beaten
>
> 1 tsp. olive oil
>
> 1/2 cup chopped red pepper

1/2 cup diced zucchini

1 small tomato

3 sprigs fresh basil (or dry)

1 clove chopped garlic

NO SALT

Put olive oil in pan; add garlic, veggies, and basil. Cook over medium heat, stirring frequently. Add egg whites and scramble until cooked.

Lunch

Tuna Salad

6 oz. water-packed tuna, drained

2 slices of tomato

1 cup romaine (or baby mixed greens)

1 cup cucumber and celery

Place salad ingredients in a bowl.

2 Tbsp. Non/low fat, low sugar dressing

OR:

4 oz. skinless chicken breast, grilled, with no oil

1 cup of vegetables

Afternoon Snack

Protein smoothie

Evening exercise

Aerobics dance class/elliptical trainer/treadmill/bike; plus 20 minutes of toning

Evening weigh in

Dinner

Tofu-Vegetable Stir-Fry

1 oz. extra firm tofu, cubed

1 cup vegetables (bell peppers, mushrooms, onion, broccoli)

1 garlic clove

1/4 Tbsp. red pepper flakes

Spray wok or nonstick skillet with nonfat cooking spray. Sauté red pepper flakes on medium-high heat; add garlic, onion, and vegetables. Cook for 2–3 minutes, add tofu and stir-fry until heated through.

OR:

4 oz. protein from list

1 cup vegetables

Evening Snack – optional

Unsalted microwave oil-free popcorn

Cherry tomatoes and cucumber slices with fat-free dressing dip, if desired

Day Nine

"In truth the only difference between those who have failed and those who have succeeded lies in the difference of their habits." – Og Mandino

Action Step

Take Action by Eliminating the "Try."

Often, we talk to ourselves and others using the word "try" rather than "will." Have you ever heard yourself saying "I'll try to eat healthy," or "I'll try to work out," or "I'll try to drink more water"? Watch how you talk to yourself and others about your fitness goals and habits. Use the words "I will" and "I am," and follow up with actions that align affirmative words with positive behavior. These habits will become your routine and success will breed more success.

Step One

Stay On Track

Keep with the plan, focus on your goal.

Step Two

Stay Positive

1. Take a minute to give yourself an ego boost. Repeat some motivational words out loud or to yourself.

2. Avoid negative talk, such as "I'm not good at this" or "I can't do it."

3. Remind yourself that you deserve happiness and you ARE making positive changes.

Step Three

Get support. Tell your friends and family about your healthy habits!

Morning weigh in

Morning exercise

Breakfast or Mid-morning Meal

1 cup oatmeal

2 slices turkey bacon or 2 soy sausage links

OR:

Whey protein shake (see Day Eight)

Lunch

Bun-free burger

> 1 extra lean patty
>
> 2 oz. low-fat cheese
>
> 4 leaves green lettuce
>
> 1 Tbsp. mustard
>
> Cook patty with cheese on top, place on lettuce.

OR:

Spinach salad

> 1 cup fresh spinach
>
> 1 hardboiled egg
>
> 3 oz. sliced grilled chicken breast
>
> 1 cup shredded vegetables
>
> 1/2 cup sliced mushrooms

2 Tbsp. low-fat dressing

Afternoon Snack

Protein smoothie

Evening exercise

Aerobics dance class/elliptical trainer/treadmill/bike; plus 20 minutes of toning

Evening weigh in

Dinner

Beef Tenderloin and Mashed Cauliflower

> 4 oz. grilled beef tenderloin

1 cup mixed salad greens

2 Tbsp. low-cal dressing

1 medium head cauliflower, cut into florets

1 cup purified water

2 garlic cloves, minced

1 tsp. fresh chives, chopped

1/2 tsp. onion powder

1/2 tsp. fresh parsley, chopped

1 Tbsp. chicken broth

In a medium pot, place cauliflower with water and bring to a quick boil. Lower heat to simmer and cover. Cook for an additional 12 minutes or until soft. Drain; transfer cauliflower to a bowl and mash. Blend in garlic, chives, onion powder, parsley, and broth with the mashed cauliflower. Serve hot.

OR:

4 oz. protein from option list

1 cup vegetables

Evening Snack – optional

Baked/toasted tortilla and salsa

Day Ten

"If you want your future to be different than your past study your past." – Baruch
Spinoza

Action Step

Step One

Write down three negative beliefs that have kept you from achieving your health/fitness goals.

Step Two

Write down three actions you are taking NOW to eliminate these limiting thoughts.

Step Three

Write down three ways your life will improve after you are free of the negative beliefs.

Move forward from this day empowered with a new understanding of who you are becoming, knowing you are moving closer and closer to your fitness goals!

Example:

Step One

1) I can't change my body.

2) I don't like to exercise.

3) I like to eat junk food.

Step Two

1) I'm losing weight.

2) I enjoy how strong I feel when I exercise.

3) I am in control of everything I eat.

Step Three

1) I will feel and look wonderful!

2) I will feel strong and healthy, and excited to take on new challenges.

3) I will be proud that I take care of my body and appreciate my great health.

Morning weigh in

Morning exercise

Breakfast or Mid-morning Meal

Whey protein shake (see Day Eight)

OR:

Omelet with Cheese

> 6 egg whites
>
> 2 Tbsp. red and/or green bell pepper
>
> 1 Tbsp. scallions
>
> 2 Tbsp. reduced fat cheese
>
> Spray nonstick cooking pan with cooking spray. Add pepper and scallions. Pour in egg whites. Add cheese. Fold.

Lunch

3 oz. slices of turkey, chicken, or tofu

4 leaves of lettuce

1/2 bell pepper, cut into strips

1 tsp. reduced fat mayo, mustard, or 1 Tbsp. reduced fat salad dressing

Place meat on lettuce, spread with mayo, and roll it up.

OR:

Grilled or Baked Chicken Salad

> 3 oz. Grilled or baked chicken
>
> 2 cup lettuce
>
> 1/2 cup vegetables
>
> 2 Tbsp. low-cal dressing

Afternoon Snack

Protein smoothie

Evening exercise

Aerobics dance class/elliptical trainer/treadmill/bike; plus 20 minutes of toning

Evening weigh in

Dinner

Lemon Chicken Breast

1 skinless boneless chicken thigh

Lemon juice

1 shallot

1/2 Tbsp. capers

1 Tbsp. Dijon mustard

1 cup steamed vegetables

Place the chicken in a shallow roasting pan and cover with the sauce. Broil for 12–15 minutes until chicken is fully cooked.

OR:

4 oz. protein from option list

1 cup vegetables

Evening Snack – optional

Four extra lean ham slices topped with mustard

Raw vegetables (celery sticks, baby carrots, broccoli, etc.) with fat-free dressing dip, if desired

Day Eleven

*"Mind, body and spirit act in concert to determine health and well being." – Dr.
Carl Thoresen*

Action Step

Focus on your well-being. Health is a state of complete physical, mental, and social well-being, and not merely the absence of disease or infirmity.

Keeping track of your waist measurement is an easy way to measure the progress that you are making. The recommended waist measurement for women is 32" or less, and the healthy waist measurement for a man is 35" or less.

Morning weigh in

Morning exercise

Breakfast or Mid-morning Meal

Salmon Scramble

2 eggs or 6 egg whites

1 oz. smoked salmon, cut in thin strips

1 Tbsp. chives or other herbs, to taste

Heat nonfat cooking spray in nonstick pan over medium heat for 1 minute. Add eggs, salmon, and herbs.

OR:

1 cup oatmeal

2 slices turkey bacon or 2 soy sausage links

Lunch

Grilled Hamburger Patty on Lettuce

1 extra lean hamburger patty

2 cups lettuce

2 Tbsp. nonfat dressing

1 cup vegetables

OR:

Tofu Salad

      1/2 cup firm tofu, cubed

      2 cups mixed green salad

      1/2 vegetables

      1 tsp. sesame seeds

      2 Tbsp. nonfat dressing

Afternoon Snack

Protein smoothie

Evening exercise

Aerobics dance class/elliptical trainer/treadmill/bike; plus 20 minutes of toning

Evening weigh in

Dinner

Whey protein shake (see Day Eight)

OR:

4 oz. protein from option list

1 cup vegetables

Evening Snack – optional

Four rolled turkey slices with/without mustard

Cherry tomatoes and cucumber slices with fat-free dressing dip, if desired

Day Twelve

"Many of life's failures are people who did not realize how close they were to success when they gave up." – Thomas Edison

Action Step

Use your positive progress to push forward.

1. Be sure to celebrate your accomplishments during your program. Be proud of yourself for all your hard work, for better food choices, and even for drinking that extra sip of water.

2. Refuse to put down or belittle yourself. Don't dwell on the things you didn't do perfectly this week. Choose to move forward instead of remaining stuck in the past.

3. Reward yourself and take time to enjoy one of your favorite activities – reading a good book, taking a hot bath, going to a movie, taking a nap, going out with family and friends, getting a manicure, a pedicure, a massage, or anything that satisfies your soul.

Morning weigh in

Morning exercise

Breakfast or Mid-morning Meal

Egg white omelet (see Day Eight)

OR:

Whey protein shake (see Day Eight)

Lunch

Ham or Turkey Sandwich

> 1 whole wheat pita
>
> 3 oz. lean ham or turkey
>
> Mustard
>
> 1 Tbsp. reduced fat mayo
>
> 3 leaves romaine lettuce

OR:

Better BOCABurger

    BOCA or veggie burger

    1 whole wheat toasted bun

    1 Tbsp. olive oil

    2 slices of tomato

    3 leaves of lettuce

    1 slice red onion

Afternoon Snack

Protein smoothie

Evening exercise

Aerobics dance class/elliptical trainer/treadmill/bike; plus 20 minutes of toning

Evening weigh in

Dinner

Salmon & Vegetables

1 salmon fillet, grilled with nonfat cooking spray for 8 –10 minutes

1 cup steamed vegetables

OR:

4 oz. protein from option list

1 cup vegetables

Evening Snack – optional

Baked/toasted tortilla and salsa

Day Thirteen

"Appreciation can make a day, even change a life. Your willingness to put it into words is all that is necessary." – Margaret Cousins

Action Step

Start a Gratitude Journal

Sarah Breathnach describes the benefits of keeping a Gratitude Journal in her book, *Simple Abundance*. She states that a Gratitude Journal can "change the quality of your life beyond belief."

Before you go to sleep, record five things you are grateful for. Your outlook on life will change as you continue to keep your gratitude journal, because you will be looking for the things you are thankful for each day and recording them later in your journal. This process produces positive results in all areas of one's life, including the area of health and fitness.

When recording what you are grateful for, be conscious of noting feelings of gratitude that are affecting your physical body and health.

Examples could be "I am grateful for drinking 10 glasses of water today to cleanse my body, I am grateful for how strong I feel, I am grateful for the long walk/run I took today, I am grateful for the people who support my health, I am grateful for making good food choices at the restaurant today, or simply I am grateful for my body."

Morning weigh in

Morning exercise

Breakfast or Mid-morning Meal

1 cup oatmeal

2 slices turkey bacon or 2 soy sausage links

OR:

Whey protein shake (see Day Eight)

Lunch

Tuna Salad

6 oz. water-packed tuna, drained

2 slices of tomato

1 cup romaine (or baby mixed greens)

1 cup cucumber and celery

Place salad ingredients in a bowl. Add 1/2 tsp. relish; mix tuna, mayo, and celery.

2 tbsp. low fat dressing

OR:

Roll Ups

3 oz. sliced turkey, ham, chicken, or tofu

4 leaves of lettuce

1/2 bell pepper, cut into strips

1 tsp. reduced fat mayo, mustard, or 1 Tbsp. reduced fat salad dressing

Place meat on lettuce, spread with mayo, and roll it up.

Afternoon Snack

Protein smoothie

Evening exercise

Aerobics dance class/elliptical trainer/treadmill/bike; plus 20 minutes of toning

Evening weigh in

Dinner

Steak & Broccoli

4–6 oz. lean filet or sirloin steak

1 tsp. olive oil

Brush the steak with the oil on sides, then grill or barbecue to taste.

1 cup steamed broccoli

OR:

4 oz. protein from option list

1 cup vegetables

Evening Snack – optional

Four rolled turkey slices with/without mustard

Raw vegetables (celery sticks, baby carrots, broccoli, etc.) with fat-free dressing dip, if desired

Day Fourteen

"First we form habits, then they form us. Conquer your bad habits, or they'll eventually conquer you." – Ancient Proverb

Action Step

Recognize your progress and recommit. Acknowledge all of the changes you've made along the way. Write down all the things that have improved for you. Do you have more energy? Have you lost pounds and inches? Are you eating healthier? Has the way you look at your health changed? Large or small, all improvements matter.

Evaluate your progress. Only you know if you can "raise the bar" and push yourself more to achieve the goals you have set for yourself. As you progress through your program, look at your goals again and recommit yourself to positive change. You are on the right path! Remind yourself of where you are going and what it takes to get there!

Morning weigh in

Morning exercise

Breakfast or Mid-morning Meal

Coffee/tea/or personal choice

Egg white omelet (see Day Eight)

OR:

Whey protein shake (see Day Eight)

Lunch

Turkey Sandwich

> 1 whole wheat pita
>
> 3 oz. lean turkey
>
> Mustard
>
> 1 Tbsp. reduced fat mayo
>
> 3 leaves of romaine

OR:

Tofu Salad

>1/2 cup firm tofu, cubed

>2 cups mixed green salad

>1/2 vegetables

>1 tsp. sesame seeds

>2 Tbsp. nonfat dressing

Afternoon Snack

Protein smoothie

Evening exercise

Aerobics dance class/elliptical trainer/treadmill/bike; plus 20 minutes of toning

Evening weigh in

Dinner

Chicken Breast and Vegetables

4 oz. skinless boneless chicken breast baked with seasoning

1 cup green beans or other vegetable

OR:

4 oz. protein from option list

1 cup vegetables

Evening Snack – optional

Unsalted microwave oil-free popcorn

Cherry tomatoes and cucumber slices with fat-free dressing dip, if desired

Day Fifteen

"While we may not be able to control all that happens to us, we can control what happens inside us." – Ben Franklin

Action Step

Practice eating mindfully. Consider the following suggestions:

Breathe deeply and relax before you eat.

Eat sitting down.

Eat without TV, newspaper, or computer.

Chew your food 30–50 times per bite.

Eating while multitasking, driving, working through lunch or watching TV often leads us to eat more than we realize. On the other hand, eating "mindfully," savoring every mouthful, enhances the experience of eating and keeps us aware of how much we take in. Stephanie Vangsness, R.D., L.D.N., C.N.S.D., author of the article "Mindful Eating," www.intelihealth.com describes this behavior as follows: "…66% of Americans report regularly eating dinner in front of the television. With obesity at epidemic proportions, it is essential that we look at not just what we eat, but how we eat."

"Scientists are beginning to evaluate and better understand the complex role of the mind-body connection in eating behavior. It turns out that when our mind is tuned out during mealtime, the digestive process may be 30% to 40% less effective. This can contribute to digestive distress, such as gas, bloating and bowel irregularities.   Gas and bloating aside, overeating and obesity are perhaps the most significant health problems caused, at least in part, by mindless eating."

"The mind-body connection plays a pivotal role in our ability to accurately assess hunger and fullness.   While the precise mechanisms of hunger and fullness are not completely understood, we do know that the brain and central nervous system receive signals from the body when food is desired or needed.   These signals can be caused by many triggers, including psychological states such as our mood."

"Once eating is under way, the brain has a key role to send out a signal when fullness is approaching. If the mind is 'multi-tasking' during eating, critical signals that regulate food intake may not be received by the brain. If the brain does not receive certain messages that occur during eating, such as sensation of taste and satisfaction, it may fail to register the event as 'eating.' This scenario can lead to the brain's continuing to send out additional signals of hunger, increasing the risk of overeating."

Morning weigh in

Morning exercise

Breakfast or Mid-morning Meal

Coffee/tea/or personal choice

Blended smoothie with 1–2 scoops protein powder

OR:

1 cup oatmeal

1/2 cup skim milk or soy milk

2 slices turkey bacon or 2 soy sausage links

1 fruit

Lunch

6-8 oz grilled skinless chicken breast

Steamed broccoli and cauliflower

Iced tea/natural low calorie soda

Afternoon Snack

Protein smoothie

Evening exercise

Aerobics dance class/elliptical trainer/treadmill/bike; plus 20 minutes of toning

Evening weigh in

Dinner

6-8 oz grilled salmon

Steamed vegetables

Sparkling mineral water/iced tea/water

Evening Snack – optional

Four extra lean ham slices topped with mustard

Raw vegetables (celery sticks, baby carrots, broccoli, etc.) with fat-free dressing dip, if desired

Day Sixteen

"Virtually nothing on earth can stop a person with a positive attitude who has their goal clearly in sight." – Denis Waitley

Action Step

Positive thinking + Positive action = Success

Choose one specific fitness goal and create a "WISH- DO- HAVE" equation.

"WISH" + "DO" = "HAVE"

"Wish" is your goal.

"Do" is your focused action.

"Have" is your positive result actualized.

Morning weigh in

Morning exercise

Breakfast or Mid-morning Meal

Coffee/tea/or personal choice

Blended smoothie with 1–2 scoops protein powder

OR:

Egg white omelet with salsa

6 oz. vegetable juice

Lunch

6-8 oz roasted skinless turkey breast

Mixed salad with fat-free dressing, if needed, or steamed vegetables

Iced tea/natural low calorie soda

Afternoon Snack

Protein smoothie

Evening exercise

Aerobics dance class/elliptical trainer/treadmill/bike; plus 20 minutes of toning

Evening weigh in

Dinner

6-8 oz grilled halibut

Steamed vegetables

Sparkling mineral water/iced tea/water

Evening Snack – optional

Baked/toasted tortilla and salsa

Day Seventeen

Dance like nobody's watching.

Action Step

Congratulate yourself each day knowing that you're not only increasing your aerobic capacity, you are also improving your dancing skills. Pride yourself on the fact that you're developing a new a new talent and building hand/eye and foot/eye coordination.

Don't worry about whether you're doing the movements "right," just keep moving and have fun.

Morning weigh in

Morning exercise

Breakfast or Mid-morning Meal

Coffee/tea/or personal choice

Blended smoothie with 1–2 scoops protein powder

OR:

Scrambled egg whites with peppers and onions

6 oz. vegetable juice

Lunch

6-8 oz lean steak

Steamed broccoli and cauliflower

Iced tea/natural low calorie soda

Afternoon Snack

Protein smoothie

Evening exercise

Aerobics dance class/elliptical trainer/treadmill/bike; plus 20 minutes of toning

Evening weigh in

Dinner

6-8 oz grilled haddock

Steamed cauliflower

Sparkling mineral water/iced tea/water

Evening Snack – optional

Four rolled turkey slices with/without mustard

Cherry tomatoes and cucumber slices with fat-free dressing dip, if desired

Day Eighteen

"Habit simplifies the movements required to achieve a given result, make them more accurate and diminish fatigue." – Ashleigh Brilliant

Action Step

Drink More Water

Are you drinking enough? If you feel thirsty, you are already dehydrated. Drink a glass of water with each meal and between each meal. Hydrate before, during, and after exercise. Substitute sparkling water for alcoholic drinks at social gatherings.

Body Benefits: Drinking more water results in weight loss.

Dehydration can slow your metabolism. Water is your body's principal chemical component, comprising, on average, 60 percent of your weight. Every system in your body depends on water. Water flushes toxins out of vital organs, carries nutrients to your cells, and provides a moist environment for ear, nose, and throat tissues.

Morning weigh in

Morning exercise

Breakfast or Mid-morning Meal

Coffee/tea/or personal choice

Blended smoothie with 1–2 scoops protein powder

OR:

Egg white omelet (see Day Eight)

1 slice whole wheat toast with 1 tsp. light butter (such as Smart Balance)

6 oz. vegetable juice

Lunch

4 oz lean hamburger with mustard, lettuce, tomato, and onion, without the bun

Iced tea/natural low calorie soda

Afternoon Snack

Protein smoothie

Evening exercise

Aerobics dance class/elliptical trainer/treadmill/bike; plus 20 minutes of toning

Evening weigh in

Dinner

6-8 oz baked skinless chicken breast

Steamed vegetables

Sparkling mineral water/iced tea/water

Evening Snack – optional

Baked/toasted tortilla and salsa

Day Nineteen

"Discipline is remembering what you want." – David Campbell

Action Step

It takes discipline to say no time and again to friends, family, and co-workers offering you unhealthy food or unhealthy choices. Work on creating an automatic response, something you will say when someone offers you something you don't want to eat or suggests an activity that takes you away from your healthy lifestyle.

Why does it seem that people close to you go out of their way to sabotage you?

Getting fit through diet and exercise takes discipline. When we create changes in our life, some of these changes may affect our family, friends, and even co-workers. If your family and friends are supportive of your healthy lifestyle, let them know how much you appreciate their positive reinforcement; but if they're not supportive, they actually may be uncomfortable with your plan and (unintentionally) sabotage it.

Morning weigh in

Morning exercise

Breakfast or Mid-morning Meal

Coffee/tea/or personal choice

Blended smoothie with 1–2 scoops protein powder

OR:

6–10 hardboiled egg whites

6 oz. vegetable juice

Lunch

Two-cheese (fat-free) skinless chicken breast tacos with salsa

Iced tea/natural low calorie soda

Afternoon Snack

Protein smoothie

Evening exercise

Aerobics dance class/elliptical trainer/treadmill/bike; plus 20 minutes of toning

Evening weigh in

Dinner

6-8 oz skinless Cornish hen

Mixed salad with fat-free dressing, if needed

Sparkling mineral water/tea/water

Evening Snack – optional

Unsalted microwave oil-free popcorn

Raw vegetables (celery sticks, baby carrots, broccoli, etc.) with fat-free dressing dip, if desired

Day Twenty

"Sometimes the most urgent and vital thing you can possibly do is take a complete rest." – Ashleigh Brilliant

The latest research indicates a strong link between lack of sleep and increased weight, and this may be just as crucial to shedding excess pounds as diet and regular exercise.

Sleep deprivation lowers leptin, a blood protein that suppresses appetite and seems to affect how the brain senses when the body has had enough food. Sleep deprivation also raises levels of grehlin, a substance that makes people want to eat.

Insufficient sleep has been linked with increases in fat tissue in the body and a loss of muscle strength and muscle mass. Lack of sleep causes a decrease in bone density, particularly in women, which can lead to osteoporosis.

When we are tired, we crave more sugar, caffeine, and refined carbohydrates, all of which can cause us to put on extra weight. When we do not get adequate rest, our adrenal glands are stressed and our kidneys will retain fluid, and we usually will appear puffy. If we get enough sleep, our organs will function more effectively and we will look better and appear thinner.

Americans average only a little more than six hours of sleep a night. The average adult needs eight hours of sleep a night, which means approximately nine hours in bed. People who sleep less than that have a 45% greater risk of being overweight, and those who sleep less than four hours have a 75% chance of being overweight.

Dr. Philip Eichling, a sleep and weight-loss specialist at the University of Arizona, says, "One of my treatments is to tell them [his patients] they should move from six hours to seven hours of sleep. When they're less sleepy, they're less hungry."

Action Step

Get more sleep. If your "Size 2 for Life" fitness program requires you to get up an hour earlier every day, make an adjustment and go to bed earlier each night. You can start by gradually increasing your sleep 15 minutes per night until you get at least seven hours of sleep.

Make sure to avoid caffeinated beverages later in the day which may make falling asleep more difficult.

Morning weigh in

Morning exercise

Breakfast or Mid-morning Meal

Coffee/tea/or personal choice

Blended smoothie with 1 –2 scoops protein powder

OR:

Salmon Scramble (see Day Eleven)

6 oz. vegetable juice

Lunch

6-8 oz grilled skinless chicken breast

Steamed broccoli and cauliflower

Iced tea/natural low calorie soda

Afternoon Snack

Protein smoothie

Evening exercise

Aerobics dance class/elliptical trainer/treadmill/bike; plus 20 minutes of toning

Evening weigh in

Dinner

6-8 oz broiled cod

Steamed vegetables

Sparkling mineral water/iced tea/water

Evening Snack – optional

Cherry tomatoes and cucumber slices with fat-free dressing dip, if desired

Day Twenty-One

"We are what we repeatedly do. Excellence then, is not an act, but a habit." –
Aristotle

Over the course of your program, exercise and healthy eating will become your normal habits!

Action Step

CELEBRATE YOUR SUCCESS!

Every time you drop five lbs., lose an inch, feel stronger during your workout session, or have more energy – celebrate! Do something you enjoy, and thank yourself for all of the big and small victories you achieve. You're getting healthier, stronger, and closer to reaching your goal.

ALWAYS REVISE, REASSESS, AND RECOMMIT

Look at your progress and goals, and ask yourself the following questions:

What activities am I not doing now that might help me reach my goal if I began to incorporate them into my daily life?

What obstacles still need to be overcome?

How much do I want to achieve the goal?

Is my motivation strong enough?

Are the benefits achieved worth the costs?

What is the measurable outcome?

How will I feel when I reach my desired weight and my desired level of fitness?

Do a weekly review to monitor your progress. Review the past week and create an action plan for the upcoming week. Keep up the good work, and keep thinking healthy thoughts!

Morning weigh in

Morning exercise

Breakfast or Mid-morning Meal

Coffee/tea/or personal choice

Blended smoothie with 1–2 scoops protein powder

OR:

6–10 hardboiled egg whites

6 oz. vegetable juice

Lunch

Two-cheese (fat-free) skinless chicken breast tacos with salsa

Iced tea/natural low calorie soda

Afternoon Snack

Protein smoothie

Evening exercise

Aerobics dance class/elliptical trainer/treadmill/bike; plus 20 minutes of toning

Evening weigh in

Dinner

6 oz grilled lean ham steak

Mixed salad with fat-free dressing, if needed

Sparkling mineral water/tea/water

Evening Snack – optional

Four rolled turkey slices with/without mustard

Raw vegetables (celery sticks, baby carrots, broccoli, etc.) with fat-free dressing dip, if desired

Evaluation/Reassessment Point

At this point, if you've kept to the program, you should have lost 5–15 lbs. From here, you have two choices. You can repeat the last 21-day program and continue to lose at the initial pace or greater, or you can modify the menu plan a bit and keep moving on, but at a more relaxed pace. If you're in Group #2 or higher, my suggestion is that you repeat the initial program until you're in the next lower group.

Some may want to substitute more lean chicken for the egg whites or lean red meat for some of the chicken. You may want to increase the amount of vegetables or add in a little more fruit. It's really up to you.

If you find yourself slipping back (the morning scale will tell you), then return to the start-up menu plan. But you must continue on the exercise program to really achieve your personal best.

If you haven't lost between 5–15 lbs., you need to take a critical look back at the last three weeks and acknowledge where you slacked off.

Remember the formula:

Calories expended MUST EXCEED calories consumed.

There is no way around this formula for the healthy person. If you didn't lose weight, then the inescapable fact is that you either cheated on your diet or you didn't get enough aerobic exercise to offset it.

Going to the gym and sitting around gabbing isn't exercise. Adhering to your diet and exercise program during the day and then pigging out on wine, cheese, and nuts at night isn't keeping to the program.

Only you know the answer, so only you know the solution. In any case, don't get discouraged. Making lifestyle adjustments is not as easy for some people as for others. Everyone has her /his own schedule and responsibilities and changing one's lifestyle may be a more gradual process for some than for others. If you haven't seen the kind of improvement that you should have by now, it's very simple to reevaluate and begin again. Just consider, even a one-pound drop in weight per week can lead to a 52-pound loss over the course of a year. The most important point is to not get discouraged and give up. Go back, reevaluate, and acknowledge where you cheated. Adjust your mindset and try again.

I know restating this equation is redundant and perhaps a bit irritating in its simplicity but on my personal journey to losing almost 60 pounds it was amazing how often I had to recall it. This usually came at times when I would 'plateau.' Of course, when I forced myself to address the real reasons for my lack of progress, invariably they would be ways (damn those peanuts!) in which I had fallen back on my old ways a bit and cheated. – Dr. Paulsen

From Here and Beyond

For those of you who have achieved Group #1 or who are moving along well in Group #2, there are some "sweeteners" you might want to add to your program which are not only fun and healthy, but downright addictive. One of these is Cardio Dance.

Life Long Cardio!

If your goal is to improve your fitness level and lose weight, you must get cardiovascular exercise. PERIOD! There is no "best" cardio exercise. You can walk, jog, cycle, do Cardio Dance, or perform any other aerobic activity for at least 20 minutes. The many health benefits include:

- Helps control body weight

- Helps maintain and build healthy bones, joints, and muscles

- Improves mobility

- Promotes psychological well-being

- Reduces depression

- Reduces stress and anxiety

- Increases your lung capacity

- Reduce risk of heart attack, high cholesterol, high blood pressure, and diabetes

- Improves sleep

Warning! Don't listen to the "celebrity gurus" who advocate a cardio-free workout. Their absurd assertions include: "Cardiovascular exercise kills a weight-loss plan, your internal organs, your immune system, your time and your motivation..." - *ABC News*.

This kind of gibberish may be appealing to those who want to avoid exercise and justify their unhealthy lifestyles, but the ultimate consequences could include diabetes, heart disease, osteoporosis, and more.

These gurus also neglect to point out that the key to sticking with your exercise program is making it fun! We challenge you to compare the exhilaration you feel during a cardio-intensive activity with the boring, tedious effort of trying to force yourself through an hour of an exclusively resistive routine. If you do, you'll quickly learn that these celebrity darlings are simply feeding you the misinformation they think you want to hear (so that you will buy their books). A year from now, they'll be telling you that the only exercise you need is lifting the fork to your mouth. Don't believe them! Again, *we didn't become a nation of fatties because of too much cardio.*

The truth is: You need both strength training and cardiovascular exercise if you want to lose weight and reap the psychological and physiological benefits of a healthy, trim body.

If you live in a mild climate, take it outdoors – try hiking, walking, jogging, running, or cycling. If the city you live in is seasonally too hot or too cold to comfortably exercise outdoors, you can join a gym or a local recreation center. You'll have access to stationary bikes, elliptical trainers, treadmills, rowing machines, Stairmasters, and more.

Alternatively, home exercise programs can be ideal for some. Working out at home frees you of the commute, childcare fees, and any anxiety about working out in a group class or in front of others. Depending on your current fitness level and exercise preferences, there are numerous DVDs available in every fitness genre, including dance, kickboxing, step, and Tai Chi. If you want more information and reviews about fitness DVDs, you can visit Collage Video http://www.collagevideo.com.

Cardio Dance

I've been teaching fitness and dance programs for the past fifteen years. I've taught Bootcamp, Hip Hop, Step Aerobics, Kickboxing, Salsa, '80s Dance Party, Disco Divas, On The Ball, Circuit Training, Hi Lo, Ab Lab, Ballet Buns, and my signature series, "Burn 'N Firm." I learned firsthand that people make lasting changes when they associate happiness with exercise and feeling good. When we look at our lives and think about when we were most content, it's often when we were our healthiest. I've discovered that the key to long-term success is finding a program that you truly enjoy. - Ashley

Dancing is a fun way to add variety to your cardio workouts. Not only are you burning a lot of calories, you're using every muscle in your body, improving coordination, and even improving your memory. As pointed out by Joe Verghese, M.D, et al, "Leisure Activities and the Risk of Dementia in the Elderly," *The New England Journal of Medicine*: "the only physical activity to offer protection against dementia was frequent dancing." His study demonstrated that reading led to a 35% reduced risk of dementia. Bicycling and swimming had no effect whatsoever but the protective effects of dancing were impressive.

Some people shy away from dance, thinking "I'm not a dancer, I have two left feet." But Cardio Dance is not about becoming a prima ballerina or a Latin mambo king. This is dance for fun and fitness, not a competition.

Cardio Dance classes at the gym are generally one hour, mixed level, fun, and non-competitive. You'll begin the class with a warm up, learning a few basic steps, and gradually adding more steps to create different patterns or choreography. The music, energy, and camaraderie should make you feel comfortable, even if you miss a step. In contrast, a class taken at a traditional-style dance studio where the focus is more on dance technique than cardio may leave you frustrated and sweat-less. This is not to discourage you from joining one, but you should understand that they have essentially two different purposes.

Don't be intimidated by the group of sweaty, smiling hip-shakers in the Cardio Dance class. Teaching classes, I've often had the experience of a woman coming up to me after class, beaming, and telling me that she had been watching the class for weeks as she walked on the treadmill and didn't think she could do the moves, but was so excited and had had a great time – along with a great workout! I love to see people leave the gym feeling confident, healthy, and energized.

The group dynamic is also a great motivator. So, if you've never taken any group exercise classes, give it a try – you may get hooked on a very healthy addiction. My groups of regular "Burn 'N Firmers" come to class religiously and many have developed wonderful friendships as a result of taking the class. It's more than exercise; it's a social support system, as well.

Here are a few tips if it's your first time:

- Get to class five minutes early and let the instructor know that you're new to class. Tell her/him if you have any prior injuries and ask for any modifications you may need.

- Make sure you have the right type of shoes and are wearing sportswear you can move in freely. Pants that are too tight, or forgetting to wear a good sports bra (women), can ruin the class. Usually, a cross-training shoe with good lateral/ankle support (not a jogging shoe) works well.

- Don't worry about the right, left arms up, down, turn around movements at first – the less you think about it, the easier it will be. The instructor may "cue" the move before they do it; just follow along and keep moving. If you feel lost, go back to the basic move and add on when you can.

Don't worry that anyone is watching you. Trust me, most likely they're not. Rest assured that they're totally into their own routine and oblivious to anyone else's. If they do notice you, they're probably impressed that you're trying. Remember, they were beginners once too.

Women and men of all ages have told me that the workouts fly by because of the fun moves and music, and that it's a program which creates results that last.

A useful technique for starting this or any other new venture is to accept the fact that you are a novice and are going to screw up. This way, you have no expectation of keeping up with or outperforming anyone else, and can just relax and learn. You'll be surprised at how fast you improve when you take the pressure off yourself. – Dr. Paulsen

Spinning can be a great addition to your workout routine. The beat is exhilarating, the instructors are stimulating, and the exercise is definitely cardio-active. Unfortunately, the deafening volume of the music in many of the classes is extremely harmful to the hair cells in your inner ear and can lead to permanent hearing loss. If you can find a class with an acceptable music volume or don't mind wearing ear plugs, definitely try it.

"Normalizing" Your Life

This term is really a misnomer. A normal lifestyle is a healthy lifestyle, and what you've probably been doing up until now is really better termed abnormal. Perhaps a more appropriate term would be liberalizing your lifestyle.

At this point, you should be metabolizing at a rate that allows for greater flexibility and freedom with your diet than during the start-up phases. Eating out in restaurants, at barbecues, and even having pizza and/or ice cream occasionally is no problem. Your exercise program should easily accommodate these rewards. In fact, you may find that you can eat just about anything – so long as you continue to burn off those calories. Your scale will tell you. You might even be surprised to find that eating isn't really an issue anymore.

Congratulations! You've made it. You've achieved a healthy lifestyle and can forget about dieting, just so long as you maintain your exercise program and follow the Size 2 for Life Long-term Continued Success Diet Plan.

Look in the mirror and smile. You look great and you've come a long way.

The *Size 2 for Life* Long-term Success Plan

Now that you've achieve your goal, you can feel pretty good about yourself and your new look. Maintaining a rigorous diet is no longer necessary, as long as you continue your exercise program. Eating healthy is a habit that you should embrace for life.

The following section will provide you with healthy, tasty dishes, and should help you not only maintain your new look on the outside but keep you healthy and fit on the inside. Of course, should you find yourself slipping back and packing on a few extra pounds, just return to the *Size 2 for Life* Start-up Program for a bit of a boost.

"I spent my 20's and 30s as a size 10/12 and now I'm a size 2... A couple weeks before my 41st birthday I saw a shocking family photo in which I was the largest person in the group. It made me sad and sick at the same time. I decided that lipo was the only solution for my giant belly and phoned a friend who had some success with the procedure for advice.

Her advice was blunt: "You're not going to get lipo," she said. "Instead, you're going to go on a diet and you'll lose weight.... from your arms, your legs, your butt and yes, your gut."

To prove her wrong (I couldn't possibly diet...how would I have the strength to get through the day without food?), I decided to change my relationship with food. The main thing for me was portion control. I wasn't going to deny myself anything, because as soon as I told myself that I could no longer have chocolate chip cookies, I knew that they would be the only things I would live for.

Instead, I made some simple but effective changes… I used to think that if a bite of (insert yummy food item here) tasted good and made me happy that 10 bites of (insert yummy food item here) tasted 10 times as good and made me 10 times as happy. Now, I can be happy with 1-2 bites of treats. Eating a little more slowly to enjoy the flavors longer helped.

I never thought I would see results. I always ate a lot of healthy food (emphasis on a lot) like salads, whole grains, lean meat/fish, etc., and I worked out, so I thought "this is where my adult weight is and I can't do much about it." But it was the portions that really made the difference, along with making "treat" foods like cheese, bacon, and cookies actual treats instead of a regular part of my diet.

A long time gym-goer (I was one of those fit-but-fat folks), I also upped my workouts, with a little more cardio at each visit, and an extra visit or two a week. Starting to lift weights helped too...sure, muscle weighs more than fat, but it takes up less room, so I LOOK thinner and can get into smaller clothes!

The results? I lost 20 percent of my body weight (about 30 pounds) in 6 months (slow, but sure!) and have kept the weight off for over 2 years."– Linda S.

Eat Right and Stay Slim

Most Americans consume too many calories and not enough nutrients, according to the latest revision to the Dietary Guidelines for Americans. In January 2005, two federal agencies – the Department of Health and Human Services and the Department of Agriculture (USDA) – released the guidelines to help adults and children ages two and up live healthier lives.

Currently, the typical American diet is low in fruits, vegetables, and whole grains, and high in saturated fat, salt, and sugar. As a result, more Americans than ever are overweight, obese, and at increased risk for chronic diseases such as heart disease, high blood pressure, diabetes, and certain cancers.

Of course, old habits are hard to break, and the notion of change can seem overwhelming. But it can be done with planning and a gradual approach, says Dee Sandquist, a spokeswoman for the American Dietetic Association (ADA) and manager of nutrition and diabetes at the Southwest Washington Medical Center in Vancouver, Washington.

"Some people can improve eating habits on their own, while others need a registered dietitian to guide them through the process," Sandquist says. You should definitely consider consulting a dietitian if you have a health condition such as osteoporosis, high blood pressure, high cholesterol, or diabetes.

Sandquist says that many people she counsels have been accustomed to eating a certain way, and never thought about what they were actually putting in their bodies. "Someone may tell me they drink six cans of regular soda every day," she says. "When they find out there are about nine teaspoons of sugar in one can, it puts things in perspective. Then I work with the person to cut back to three cans a day, then to two and so on, and to start replacing some of the soda with healthier options."

Sandquist says that when people strive for more balance in their diets, they tend to enjoy mixing up their food choices. "A lot of times, they've been eating the same things over and over. So when they start trying new foods, they find out what they've been missing."

Barbara Schneeman, Ph.D., director of the Food and Drug Administration's Office of Nutritional Products, Labeling, and Dietary Supplements, encourages consumers to make smart food choices from every food group. "The Nutrition Facts label is an important tool that gives guidance for making these choices," she says. The label shows how high or low a food is in various nutrients.

Experts say that once you start using the label to compare products, you'll find there is flexibility in creating a balanced diet and enjoying a variety of foods in moderation. For example, you could eat a favorite food that's higher in fat for breakfast and have lower-fat foods for lunch and dinner. You could have a full-fat dip on a low-fat cracker. "What matters is how all the food works together," Sandquist says.

Older people are most likely to improve their eating habits, but nutrition is important for people of all ages, says Walter Willet, M.D., chairman of the nutrition department at the Harvard School of Public Health. "We know that when people have health problems or their friends become ill, these are strong motivators of change," says Willet. "The more serious the health condition, the more serious the change. We'd rather people made changes early and prevent health problems in the first place."

Here are some tips to keep your eating habits moving in the right direction.

Look at What You Eat Now

Look for healthier versions of what you like to eat. If you like luncheon meat sandwiches, try a reduced-fat version. If you like the convenience of frozen dinners, look for ones with lower sodium. If you love fast-food meals, try a salad as your side dish instead of french fries.

Use the Nutrition Facts Label

To make smart food choices quickly and easily, compare the Nutrition Facts labels on products. Look at the Percent Daily Value (%DV) column. The general rule of thumb is that 5 percent or less of the Daily Value is considered low and 20 percent or more is high.

Keep saturated fat, trans fat, cholesterol, and sodium low, while keeping fiber, potassium, iron, calcium, and vitamins A and C high. Be sure to look at the serving size and the number of servings per package. The serving size affects calories, amounts of each nutrient, and the percentage of Daily Value.

The %DV is based on a 2,000-calorie diet, but recommended calorie intake differs for individuals based on age, gender, and activity level. Some people need less than 2,000 calories a day. You can use the %DV as a frame of reference whether or not you consume more or less than 2,000 calories. The %DV makes it easy to compare the nutrients in each food product to see which ones are higher or lower. When comparing products, just make sure the serving sizes are similar, especially the weight (grams, milligrams, or ounces) of each product.

Control Portion Sizes

Understanding the serving size on the Nutrition Facts label is important for controlling portions, Someone may have a large bottled drink and assume it's only one serving. But if you look at the label, it's actually two servings. If you consume two servings of a product, you have to multiply all the numbers by two. When the servings go up, so do the calories, fat, sugar, and salt.

Try dishing out a smaller amount on your plate, or use smaller plates. If you put more food in front of you, you'll eat it because it's there. According to the ADA, an average serving size of meat looks like a deck of cards. An average serving size of pasta or rice is about the size of a tennis ball.

Here are some other ways to limit portions: Split a meal or dessert with a friend at a restaurant, get a doggie bag for half of your meal, get in the habit of having one helping, and ask for salad dressing, butter, and sauces on the side so you can control how much you use.

Control Calories and Get the Most Nutrients

"You want to stay within your daily calorie needs, especially if you're trying to lose weight," says Eric Hentges, Ph.D., director of the USDA Center for Nutrition Policy and Promotion. "But you also want to get the most nutrients out of the calories, which means picking nutritionally rich foods," he says. Children and adults should pay particular attention to getting adequate calcium, potassium, fiber, magnesium, and vitamins A, C, and E.

According to the Dietary Guidelines, there is room for what's known as a discretionary calorie allowance. This is for when people meet their recommended nutrient intake without using all their calories. Hentges compares the idea to a household budget. "You know you have to pay all the bills and then you can use the leftover money for other things," he says. "The discretionary calorie allowance gives you some flexibility to have foods and beverages with added fats and sugars, but you still want to make sure you're getting the nutrients you need." For example, a 2,000-calorie diet has about 250 discretionary calories, according to the Dietary Guidelines.

Know Your Fats

Fat provides flavor and makes you feel full. It also provides energy, and essential fatty acids for healthy skin, and helps the body absorb the fat-soluble vitamins A, D, E, and K. But fat also has nine calories per gram, compared to four calories per gram in carbohydrates and protein. If you eat too much fat every day, you may get more calories than your body needs, and too many calories can contribute to weight gain.

Too much saturated fat, trans fat, and cholesterol in the diet increases the risk of unhealthy blood cholesterol levels, which may increase the risk of heart disease.

"Consumers should lower all three, not just one or the other," says Schneeman. Saturated fat is found mainly in foods from animals. Major sources of saturated fats are cheese, beef, and milk. Trans fat results when manufacturers add hydrogen to vegetable oil to increase the food's shelf life and flavor. Trans fat can be found in vegetable shortenings, some margarines, crackers, cookies, and other snack foods. Cholesterol is a fat-like substance in foods from animal sources such as meat, poultry, egg yolks, milk, and milk products.

Most of your fats should come from polyunsaturated and monounsaturated fatty acids, such as those that occur in fish, nuts, soybean, corn, canola, olive, and other vegetable oils. This type of fat does not raise the risk of heart disease and may be beneficial when consumed in moderation.

Make Choices That Are Lean, Low-fat, or Fat-free

When buying meat, poultry, milk, or milk products, choose versions that are lean, low-fat, or fat-free. Choose lean meats like chicken without the skin, and lean beef or pork with the fat trimmed off.

If you frequently drink whole milk, switch to 1 percent milk or skim milk. Many people don't taste a difference. Some mix whole milk with lower-fat milk for a while so the taste buds can adjust. "This doesn't mean you can never eat or drink the full-fat versions," Schneeman says. "That's where the discretionary calories come in."

Other tips to reduce saturated fat include cooking with nonstick sprays and using olive, safflower, or canola oils instead of lard or butter. Eat more fish, which is usually lower in saturated fat than meat. Bake, grill, and broil food instead of frying it because more fat is absorbed into the food when frying. You could also try more meatless entrees like veggie burgers, and add flavor to food with a low-fat bean spread instead of butter.

Focus on Fruit

The Dietary Guidelines recommend two cups of fruit per day at the 2,000-calorie reference diet. Fruit intake and recommended amounts of other food groups vary at different calorie levels. An example of two cups of fruit includes: one small banana, one large orange, and one-fourth cup of dried apricots or peaches.

Eat a variety of fruits – whether fresh, frozen, canned, or dried – rather than fruit juice for most of your fruit choices. "The whole fruit has more fiber, it's more filling, and it's naturally sweet," says Marilyn Tanner, a pediatric dietitian at the Washington University School of Medicine in St. Louis. Still, some juices, such as orange and prune, are a good source of potassium.

Ways to incorporate fruit in your diet include adding it to your cereal, eating it as a snack with low-fat yogurt or a low-fat dip, or making a fruit smoothie for dessert by mixing low-fat milk with fresh or frozen fruit such as strawberries or peaches. Also, your family is more likely to eat fruit if you put it out on the kitchen table.

Eat Your Veggies

The Dietary Guidelines recommend two and one-half cups of vegetables per day if you eat 2,000 calories each day.

Tanner suggests adding vegetables to foods such as meatloaf, lasagna, omelets, stir-fry dishes, and casseroles. Frozen chopped greens such as spinach, and peas, carrots, and corn are easy to add. Also, add dark leafy green lettuce to sandwiches. "Involve kids by letting them help pick vegetables in different colors when you're shopping," Tanner suggests. Get a variety of dark green vegetables such as broccoli, spinach, and greens; orange and deep yellow vegetables such as carrots, winter squash, and sweet potatoes; starchy vegetables like corn; legumes, such as dry beans, peas, chickpeas, pinto beans, kidney beans, and tofu; and other vegetables, such as tomatoes and onions.

"Look for ways to make it convenient," Tanner says. "You can buy salad in a bag. Or, buy a vegetable tray from the grocery store and put it in the refrigerator. Everything's already cut up and you can just reach in and eat it throughout the week."

Make Half Your Grains Whole

Like fruits and vegetables, whole grains are a good source of vitamins, minerals, and fiber. The Dietary Guidelines recommend at least three ounces of whole grains per day. One slice of bread, one cup of breakfast cereal, or one-half cup of cooked rice or pasta are each equivalent to about one ounce. Tanner suggests baked whole-grain corn tortilla chips or whole-grain cereal with low-fat milk as good snacks.

In general, at least half the grains you consume should come from whole grains. For many, but not all, whole grain products, the words "whole" or "whole grain" will appear before the grain ingredient's name. The whole grain must be the first ingredient listed in the ingredients list on the food package. The following are some whole grains: whole wheat, whole oats or oatmeal, whole-grain corn, popcorn, wild rice, brown rice, buckwheat, whole rye, bulgur or cracked wheat, whole-grain barley, and millet. Whole-grain foods cannot necessarily be identified by their color or by names such as brown bread, nine-grain bread, hearty grains bread, or mixed grain bread.

Lower Sodium and Increase Potassium

Higher salt intake is linked to higher blood pressure, which can raise the risk of stroke, heart disease, and kidney disease. The Dietary Guidelines recommend that people consume less than 2,300 milligrams of sodium per day (approximately one teaspoon of salt). There are other recommendations for certain populations that tend to be more sensitive to salt. For example, people with high blood pressure, blacks, and middle-aged and older adults should consume no more than 1,500 milligrams of sodium each day.

Most of the sodium people eat comes from processed foods. Use the Nutrition Facts label on food products: 5%DV or less for sodium means the food is low in sodium, and 20%DV or more means it's high. Compare similar products and choose the option with a lower amount of sodium. Most people won't notice a taste difference. Consistently consuming lower-salt products will help taste buds adapt, and you'll enjoy these foods as much or more than higher-salt options.

Prepare foods with little salt. The DASH (Dietary Approaches to Stop Hypertension) eating plan from the National Heart, Lung, and Blood Institute recommends giving flavor to food with herbs, spices, lemon, lime, vinegar, and salt-free seasoning blends. Consult with your physician before using salt substitutes because their main ingredient, potassium chloride, can be harmful to some people with certain medical conditions.

Also, increase potassium-rich foods such as sweet potatoes, orange juice, bananas, spinach, winter squash, cantaloupe, and tomato puree. Potassium counteracts some of sodium's effect on blood pressure.

Limit Added Sugars

The Dietary Guidelines recommend choosing and preparing food and beverages with little added sugars. Added sugars are sugars and syrups added to foods and beverages in processing or preparation, not the naturally occurring sugars in fruits or milk. Major sources of added sugars in the American diet include regular soft drinks, candy, cake, cookies, pies, and fruit drinks. In the ingredients list on food products, sugar may be listed as brown sugar, corn syrup, glucose, sucrose, honey, or molasses. Be sure to check the sugar in low-fat and fat-free products, which sometimes contain a lot of sugar, Tanner says.

Instead of drinking regular soda and sugary fruit drinks, try natural low calorie soda, low-fat or fat-free milk, water, flavored water, or 100 percent fruit juice.

For snacks and desserts, try fruit. "People are often pleasantly surprised that fruit is great for satisfying a sweet tooth," Tanner says. "And if ice cream is calling your name, don't have it in the freezer. Make it harder to get by having to go out for it. Then it can be an occasional treat."

Smart Snacks

Applesauce
Low-fat yogurt with fruit
Unbuttered and unsalted popcorn
Broccoli, carrots, or cherry tomatoes with dip or low-fat yogurt
Grapes
Apple slices with peanut butter
Raisins
Nuts (a few)
Graham crackers
Gingersnap cookies
Low- or reduced-fat string cheese
Baked whole-grain tortilla chips with salsa
Whole-grain cereal with low-fat milk

Navigating the High-Fat Minefield

Okay, you've made the commitment to weight loss, fitness, and healthier living. Now, how do you stay with it when the world around you is committed to your failure?

Tips for Healthy Fast Food

- Look for items that are broiled or grilled; stay away from anything fried.

- Request extra tomato, onion, and lettuce.

- Ask for no cheese.

- Ask for no mayonnaise or "special" sauce.

- Ask for nonfat salad dressing or no dressing; use salsa if available.

- Look at the nutrition information to make the best fat gram or calorie choice.

Sounds easy, right? Wrong! Just try it. Decide that you're going to avoid that Big Mac and those fries. Tag along with your co-worker and head over to Burger King, KFC, etc., to pick up that salad. What do you think you'll really come back with?

As soon as you get within a block of that den of olfactory servitude, the smell of that fatty food is going to overcome you and – guaranteed – you'll be walking out with a double lard burger, jumbo fries, and shake. Sorry, but that's just the reality.

So, how do you deal with the overpowering urges passed on to you by your olfactory system? Well, the first thing you need to do is acknowledge the problem before you're confronted with it, and then try these simple suggestions from the doctor.

1) Don't go! That's right. Write down what you want and let your co-worker pick up that low-calorie, healthy lunch for you. Let them cave in to the temptation while you avoid it. One thing, though: when they bring back their jumbo fries, don't succumb to sharing them.

2) If you have to go, write down, in advance, exactly what you intend to order and have your friend order it for you. Or hand the paper to the counter attendant and let them execute it. Don't open your mouth to say a word. If you do, you're lost. Take your healthy order and walk/run away – quickly!

Unless you follow this advice devoutly, your new program is doomed to failure.

The following are some good choices. Make copies and have them available so you can just circle them when you hand them over.

Best Fast-Food Options

Subway

Order off the 6 Grams of Fat or less sub menu: lowest calorie sub is the Veggie De-lite, 230 calories, 2.5 grams fat, 37 grams carbohydrate, 7 grams protein Order off the 6 Grams of Fat or less salad menu: lowest calorie is the grilled chicken, 300 calories 3 grams of fat with fat-free Italian dressing

Baha Fresh

Mahi Mahi Ensalada

280 calories, 4 grams of fat, order with no cheese and use salsa for the dressing

Mahi Mahi Taco

177 calories, 9 grams of fat

El Pollo Loco

Flame-Broiled Skinless Chicken Breast

Order chicken skinless Calories: (155) Cholesterol: (95 mg) Fat: (4 g) Sodium: (540 mg) Exchanges: 4 Meat Protein: 29 g, Carbohydrate: 0 g, Fiber: 0 g

Pollo Choice Skinless Breast Meal

Order skinless chicken with fresh vegetables, garden salad & house salsa–use salsa as dressing, no tortilla Calories: (340) Cholesterol: (110 mg) Fat: (15 g) Sodium: Moderate (925 mg) Exchanges: 4 Meat, Bread, 2 Veg, 1 Fat Protein: 38 g, Carbohydrate: 16 g, Fiber: 6 g

BRC Burrito

Order with no rice,no cheese, add vegetables Calories: (375), Cholesterol: (15 mg) Fat: (14 g), Sodium: High (1255 mg) Exchanges: Meat, 4 Bread, 2 Fat Protein: 15 g, Carbohydrate: 60 g, Fiber: 6 g

Chicken Taco al Carbon

Calories: (135), Cholesterol: (30mg) Fat: (3 g), Sodium: (225 mg) Exchanges: 1 Meat, 1 Bread, Veg, Fat Protein: 9 g, Carbohydrate: 18 g, Fiber: 1 g

Sides

Steamed Fresh Vegetables Cal: 70, Fat: 4 g, Chol: 0, Sod: 80 mg, Prot: 3 g, Carb: 6 g, Fib: 4g Exch: 1 Veg, Fat

Pinto Beans Cal: 165, Fat: 4 g, Chol: 0, Sod: 715 mg, Prot: 8 g, Carb: 25 g, Fib: 10g Exch: Meat, 1 Br, Fat

Garden Salad Cal: 105, Fat: 7 g, Chol: 15, Sod: 135 mg, Prot: 5 g, Carb: 7 g, Fib: 1 g; Exch: Meat, Br, Veg, 1 Fat

McDonalds
Grilled Chicken Caesar Salad

100 calories, 2.5 grams fat, 3 grams carbohydrate, 17 grams protein, 1 vegetable exchange and 2 very lean meat exchanges. Choose one of the fat-free or reduced fat dressings.

Burger King
Chicken Whopper Jr.

344 calories, 14 grams fat, 31 grams carbohydrates, 23 grams protein. Exchanges: 3 starch, 2.75 meat (very lean). Without mayo: deduct 9 grams fat and 80 calories.

Whopper Jr.

Order without mayo or cheese: 317 calories, 13 grams fat, 32 grams carbohydrate, 16 grams protein. Exchanges: 1.75 starch, 2 meat

Chicken Caesar Salad (no croutons)

220 calories, 5 grams carbohydrate, 7 grams fat, 3 grams fiber, 35 grams protein, no trans fat. With Italian Lite dressing, add 4 grams carbohydrate, 5 grams fat, 50 calories.

Side Garden Salad

25 calories, 5 grams carbohydrate, 2 grams fiber, 0 fat, 1 gram protein

Wendy's
Grilled Chicken Sandwich

300 calories, 8 grams fat, 36 grams carbohydrate, 24 grams protein. Exchanges: 2 starch, 3 very lean meat, 1/2 high-fat meat.

Small Chili

227 calories, 7 grams fat, 21 grams carbohydrate, 15 grams protein, 5 grams fiber. Exchanges: 2 starch, 1 high-fat meat, 1 very lean meat

Caesar Side Salad (no dressing or croutons)

70 calories, 4 grams fat, 2 grams carbohydrate, 7 grams protein, 45% Vitamin A, 30% Vitamin C. Use the Fat Free French dressing (80 calories, 19 grams carbohydrates, 0 fat) or one of the reduced fat dressings. For those on a low carb diet, the Caesar dressing is the best option, it adds only 1 gram of carbohydrate, has 16 grams fat, 150 calories

Ordering At a Restaurant

Choose items that are prepared by low-fat methods – steamed, broiled, baked, grilled, stir-fried.

Eat a salad chock-full of vegetables without dressing with your meal – or better yet, order steamed vegetable so you can avoid the "fatty dressing challenge" altogether.

If you order a salad, ask for low-fat dressing on the side, or just add balsamic vinegar.

Skip the bread.

Grilled fish or chicken with steamed vegetables is a great choice.

Don't overeat! Use portion control!

You can check the nutritional value of almost everything at: www.calorieking.com

Size 2 Your Driving

Perhaps the single biggest culprit in the decline of our health and the expansion of our waistlines is the internal combustion engine. Prior to the invention of the automobile, if a person wanted to move something (including their fat asses) from one place to another, they had to provide the energy required to accomplish that goal. Today this is all done routinely by the car. Additional consequences, of course, include the heating up of our environment, the pollution of the air we breathe, and all the consequences that go along with it.

One of the most pathetic anecdotes of our current lifestyle is the one about the gym member who lives within walking distance of the gym, but chooses to drive there anyway.

She searches diligently for the closest parking space, and then goes in and spends most of the one-hour "workout" with her trainer in minimal calorie-burning yapping about the congestion on the freeways or her poodle's heart disease. Of course, after the "workout," it's back in the car for a two-block trip over to Mega Burger. Total calories expended with her trainer: 125. Total calories consumed after such a "commendable" workout: upwards of 1250.

We've become a society addicted to our cars – and it shows. If you think I'm kidding, the next time you're at the mall, take a look around at the people there. The odds are pretty good that a large majority of them will be overweight, or even obese, and they won't be walking, they'll be waddling. That's what happens when you take walking out of your daily routine. You start to gain weight, and then you exercise even less. And since you continue to eat, the cycle gets worse as the weight gain intensifies.

For some reason, people seem obligated to drive everywhere these days. No one would ever think about walking more than a few blocks. That idea seems absurd; why walk when you can drive? But that is exactly the kind of mentality that is causing people of all ages, all across the country, to continue their love affair with the automobile.

You can burn an extra 300–1000 cal/day just walking. Driving to the store will burn about 50 calories. Walking will burn around 250. Same goes for all your little chores. Hey, no one is asking you to lug huge bags of groceries, but for small items, or those that fit in a cart, choose to walk instead of drive. The benefit will add up over time.

Sedentary Life Can Be Deadly

New studies are showing that a sedentary lifestyle can result in muscle loss and significantly lowered aerobic capacity.

Researchers at the Department of Physical Education at San Diego State University recently completed a 23-year study involving two groups of middle-aged men. One group exercised regularly for 23 years. The other exercised approximately five years and then stopped.

At the end of the study, when researchers tested the fitness of the men, they found those who hadn't exercised had lost 41 percent of their maximal aerobic power, while those who exercised lost only 13 percent. These results were interesting, since decreased aerobic power has long been thought to be a natural product of aging.

Additionally, the researchers found that none of the men in the exercise group developed high blood pressure, although two men in this group had high blood pressure initially. In contrast, 60 percent of the men who didn't exercise developed high blood pressure.

Another health bonus the researchers discovered was that the blood pressure of the men who exercised was 25 percent below the average for men their age.

The long-term health benefits from walking include:

Lower blood pressure. Exercise causes blood vessels to dilate, which reduces the pressure on blood vessel walls. Decreased pressure lowers the chance of a blood vessel rupturing in the brain, thus lowering the risk for a stroke.

Lower cholesterol. Exercise lowers your cholesterol level, which decreases the risk to your heart.

Strengthened heart and cardiovascular system. The elevated heart rate you get from walking will help lower your resting heart rate. A strengthened heart and cardiovascular system also lowers the risk of coronary disease and heart attack.

Increased bone density. As density increases, the risk of osteoporosis and bone fractures decreases. Weight-bearing exercise, such as walking, is especially important for women battling osteoporosis.

Production of growth hormones that counteract the effects of aging. As you grow older, your body stops producing hormones that help keep muscles strong. Therefore, regular exercise is the only natural way to get the body to continue to produce these hormones.

Increased production of endorphins. Endorphins improve mental and physical health, and are the body's natural way to decrease stress, helping you to relax. Forty minutes of walking three to four times a week can reduce depression and anxiety. As a result of endorphin release, people often find they feel better and sleep more soundly.

Weight loss or weight maintenance. Studies have shown that walking regularly can help you lose weight and keep unwanted pounds from returning. Depending on your pace, a one-mile walk burns approximately 100 calories for a person of average weight, and perhaps more for a heavier person (up to 300 calories per hour).

Strengthened nervous system and reflexes. When your body moves, the brain sends messages to muscles that tell the muscle how to work. Those messages must be passed frequently so that the nervous system continues to function, improving your reflexes.

Increased flexibility. Walking and stretching increase overall flexibility and make daily activities, such as climbing stairs, walking across the street, and driving a car, easier and safer.

Balanced insulin production. For diabetics, exercise increases the production of insulin, which helps combat the high blood sugar of diabetes. For non-diabetics, exercise may also prevent the onset of diabetes.

With such a long list of benefits, why not start walking more and driving less? You can do it; it's never too late to get started!

Health Tips

At least 10,000 steps a day for health – and more for fitness and weight loss. Each mile walked equals about 2,000 steps.

Allow 5–10 minutes at the beginning and end of walking to warm up and cool down.

Focus on the benefits and set realistic goals.

"Life Happens" Success Strategies

Here are my ten favorite long-term "Life Happens" success strategies. When you make these habits part of your daily life, they should help you meet your fitness goals and maintain your success. - Ashley

1) Balance Your Calorie Intake
Skipping breakfast, eating chips for lunch and having a 1,200-calorie dinner only equals 1,400 calories. Perfect day? Wrong! It's not only the total number of calories consumed, but also the way you consciously spread your calories evenly throughout the day.

Aim to stay within the following calorie ranges:

- Breakfast: 300 to 500 calories

- Morning Snack: 100 to 200 calories

- Lunch: 400 to 600 calories

- Afternoon Snack: 100 to 200 calories

- Dinner: 350 to 550 calories

- Evening Snack: 50 to 150 calories

2) Eat Regularly
Women commonly make the mistake of skipping meals in an effort to lose weight. Skipping meals and snacks slows your metabolism and sets you up for binge eating. Think like an athlete in training. Food is your fuel! Avoid going long periods without eating.

For example:

7:30	a.m.	Breakfast
10:30	a.m.	Snack
12:30	p.m.	Lunch
3:00	p.m.	Snack
6:00	p.m.	Dinner
8:00	p.m.	Snack (Optional, depending on your calorie needs.)

3) Eat a Healthy Breakfast
Start each day with a healthy breakfast that provides you with 300 to 500 calories. The Size 2 for Life breakfasts will jumpstart your day and keep you satisfied. What you eat for breakfast is vital. Compare these two meal choices:

- Size <u>2</u> for Life Breakfast: Serving of oatmeal, 1/2 cup skim milk/soy milk, 2 slices turkey bacon or 2 links soy sausages/links, & 1 fruit with and a cup of tea or coffee contains only about 400 calories.

- Sugar Crash: One pastry or muffin plus cafe mocha is about 900 calories.

When you make conscious choices for breakfast, you don't only lessen your caloric intake; you also fuel yourself properly for sustained mental and physical energy.

4) Snack Smart

Snacks are an essential part of your day. Plan ahead and carry small pre-portioned bags of almonds, string cheese, and fruit or cut vegetables. Snacks are a great way to increase your intake of fruits, vegetables and fiber rich foods. Snack mid-morning and mid-afternoon.

5) Portion Control

Pay close attention to serving sizes. Remember that the portions we are commonly served in restaurants are often double or triple what they should be. Develop your awareness of portion size to practice portion control.

- 3 ounces lean meat, chicken, or fish measures looks like a deck of cards.

- 1-ounce equals about 4 dice.

- 1/2-cup pasta or rice equals an ice cream scoop.

- One fruit and vegetable serving is equal to one piece the size of a tennis ball.

6) Drink Water

The Institute of Medicine advises that women drink about 9 cups of total beverages a day. Make water your favorite beverage! Eliminate liquid calories (soda, juices, coffee drinks, sports drinks) from your day and drink water instead.

7) Limit Alcohol

Remember you are "training" like an athlete; alcohol does not support your training. Save the calories and the headaches and say "no" to alcoholic drinks and "yes" to beverages that support your health and fitness goals.

8) Eating Out can still mean Eating Right

Eating out while sticking to your healthy lifestyle is getting easier due to new legislation requiring restaurants to provide brochures with nutritional information. You can also be proactive by researching online healthy restaurants in your area.

Try some of the following tactics to help make restaurant meals fit into your healthy eating plan:

- Get exactly what you want by being specific when you order.

- Ask for healthy substitutions, for example, "I'd like a side salad instead of fries."

- Choose restaurants that have healthy items on the menu.

- Tell your sever not to bring the bread. It is easier to skip it if it's not on the table.

- Avoid items prepared with cream or other heavy sauces.

- Ask for all salad dressings on the side. Avoid bleu cheese, Caesar dressing and opt for dressing for Balsamic Vinaigrette.

- Make a meal out of healthy sided dishes like: steamed vegetables, salad, chicken breast or black beans.

- Order meats that are grilled, broiled, roasted or baked.

- Order seafood that is broiled, baked, steamed, blackened, or poached.

9) Stop Eating 3 Hours Before You Go To Bed

By imposing an eating "cut off time" of 3 (or more) hours before bed, we automatically slash our calorie intake, commonly cutting 500 to 1,000 calories per day.

10) Create a New Habit – 21-Day Transformation

Studies show that the accepted length of time to form new habits is 21 days. The best way to get rid of an unwanted habit is to replace it with a good habit for 21 consecutive days.

- Keep a Workout Log

- Use Food Journaling

- Use the "21 Tips" included in the 21-Day Program to create healthy, positive motivation for fast, lasting results.

The Size 2 for Life Real-life Meal Plan

Eating fewer calories while increasing activity is the best way to lose weight. For most adult females, a diet of 1,200– 1,500 calories per day is recommended for weight loss.

You can visit the Mayo Clinic website to determine your own daily caloric needs:

http://www.mayoclinic.com/health/calorie-calculator/NU00598

Research shows that limiting calories, not the types of foods you eat, causes more weight loss. For example, cutting only carbohydrates or fats will not cause any more weight loss than a healthful and balanced low-calorie diet.

This meal plan has approximately 1200 calories per day, including snacks. This is suitable for most women (depending on level of activity). Males and more active females need to increase the total daily calories, adding up to 600 calories by increasing the portion size or adding additional snacks from the snack option list.

GOOD MORNING!

BREAKFAST OPTIONS: (coffee or tea is acceptable)

In the Mood for Eggs

Egg White Omelet

> 6 egg whites, lightly beaten
>
> 1 tsp. olive oil
>
> 1/2 cup chopped red pepper
>
> 1/2 cup diced zucchini
>
> 1 small tomato
>
> 3 sprigs fresh basil (or dry)
>
> 1 clove chopped garlic
>
>> Put olive oil in pan; add garlic, veggies, and basil. Cook over medium heat, stirring frequently. Add egg whites and scramble until cooked.
>
> 1 slice whole wheat toast with 1 tsp. light butter (such as Earth Balance)

Simple Eggs

> Scrambled, poached, or hardboiled

> 2 pieces of lean turkey sausage or tofu sausage

> Egg whites

> 1 serving oatmeal

> 1 cup skim milk or soy milk

Salmon Scramble

> 2 eggs or 6 egg whites

> 1 oz. smoked salmon, cut in thin strips

> 1 tsp. olive oil or spray

> 1 Tbsp. chives or other herbs to taste

> Heat oil in nonstick pan over medium heat for 1 minute. Add eggs, salmon and herbs.

> 1 fruit serving

Omelet with Cheese, Please

> 6 egg whites

> 2 Tbsp. red and/or green bell pepper

> 1 Tbsp. scallions

> 2 Tbsp. reduced fat cheese

> Spray nonstick cooking pan with cooking spray. Add pepper and scallions. Pour in egg whites. Add cheese. Fold.

Yogurt and Smoothie Options

Make sure the yogurt is nonfat/PLAIN or FAGE Greek nonfat yogurt.

Yogurt Crunch with Fruit

> 8 oz. or 1 cup nonfat yogurt

> 1/2 cup sliced fresh fruit (bananas, strawberries, blueberries)

1 Tbsp. flaxseed meal

3/4 cup low-fat cereal

Mix yogurt, fruit and cereal. *Add Stevia, if needed.

Smart Smoothie

8 oz. water

1 scoop/serving soy, whey, hemp, or egg white protein powder

1 Tbsp. flaxseed meal

1 tsp. psyllium husks

1/4 cup frozen or fresh blueberries

1/2 ripe or frozen banana, or other fruit that you like

Ice (optional)

Combine all ingredients in blender. Blend until rich and creamy, about 2 to 3 minutes.

Bitter Berry Smoothie

1/4 cup cranberries, fresh or frozen

1 cup blueberries, frozen

1 scoop/serving soy, whey, hemp, or egg white protein powder

1 Tbsp. flaxseeds

Combine all ingredients in blender. Blend until rich and creamy, about 2 to 3 minutes. *Add Stevia or other no calorie sweetener, if needed.

Super Sweet Smoothie

1/2 cup skim milk or soy milk

1/2 ripe banana

1/2 can crushed pineapple

1/2 cup nonfat yogurt

1/2 scoop/serving of soy, whey, hemp, or egg white protein powder

Combine all ingredients in blender. Blend until rich and creamy, about 2 to 3 minutes.

Cereal, the Breakfast of Champions

1 cup oatmeal

1/2 cup skim milk or soy milk

2 slices turkey bacon or 2 soy sausage links

1 fruit

OR

1 cup high-fiber/low-sugar cereal (e.g., Kashi, All Bran)

1 cup skim milk or soy milk

1/2 cup fruit

Don't Like Breakfast? You Gotta Eat Something

1 slice whole wheat toast

1 tsp. almond butter, peanut butter, or light butter (such as Earth Balance)

12 almonds

1 piece fruit

LUNCHTIME OPTIONS

Salad Lovers

Tuna Salad

6 oz. water-packed tuna, drained

2 slices tomato

1 cup romaine (or baby mixed greens)

1 cup cucumber and celery

Place salad ingredients in a bowl. Add 1/2 tsp. relish; mix tuna, mayo, and celery.

2 Tbsp. Fat free low sugar dressing

4 WASA crackers

Spinach Salad

1 cup fresh spinach

1 hardboiled egg

3 oz. sliced, grilled chicken breast

1 cup shredded vegetables

1/2 cup sliced mushrooms

2 Tbsp. low-fat dressing

Greek Salad

2 cups romaine

1/2 cup tomato

1/2 cup garbanzo beans

1 Tbsp. nonfat feta cheese (Trader Joe's)

1/2 cup cucumber

1/2 Tbsp. pine nuts

2 Tbsp. nonfat dressing

Grilled Hamburger Patty on Lettuce

1 extra lean hamburger patty

2 cups lettuce

2 Tbsp. nonfat dressing

1 cup vegetables

Tofu Salad

1/2 cup firm tofu, cubed

2 cups mixed green salad

1/2 cup vegetables

1 tsp. sesame seeds

2 Tbsp. nonfat dressing

Turkey Salad

3 oz. deli turkey

2 cups green salad

3/4 cup vegetables

1 Tbsp. Fat free, low sugar dressing

4 WASA crackers

Grilled or Baked Chicken Salad

3 oz. grilled or baked chicken

2 cups lettuce

1/2 cup vegetables

2 Tbsp. low-cal dressing

4 WASA crackers

Add 1 cup or 100-calorie serving of soup (low-sodium, low-fat brand) to any of the salad options.

Tuna Sandwich

2 slices whole wheat bread

1/2 cup water-packed tuna

1 tsp. reduced fat mayo

2 Tbsp. relish

Mustard

2 slices tomato

Ham or Turkey Sandwich

1 whole wheat pita

3 oz. lean ham or turkey

Mustard

1 Tbsp. reduced fat mayo

3 leaves of romaine

Bun-Free Burger

1 extra lean meat patty

2 oz. low-fat cheese

4 leaves green lettuce

1 Tbsp. reduced fat mayo

Mustard

Cook patty with cheese on top, place on lettuce.

Better BOCA Burger

Boca or veggie burger

1 toasted whole wheat bun

1 Tbsp. olive oil

2 slices tomato

3 leaves lettuce

1 slice red onion

Roll Ups

3 oz. sliced turkey, ham, chicken, or tofu

4 leaves lettuce

1/2 bell pepper, cut into strips

1 tsp. reduced fat mayo

1 Tbsp. mustard or reduced fat salad dressing

Place meat on lettuce, spread with mayo, and roll it up.

Need a Change from Sandwiches and Salads?

More Lunch Options

Chicken Kabob

> 4 oz. cooked chicken
>
> 1/2 cup green, red, or yellow bell pepper
>
> 5 cherry tomatoes
>
> 3 large mushrooms
>
> Cut into pieces and put on skewer.

Taco

> 3 oz. lean ground beef, cooked and seasoned
>
> 1/4 cup cooked pinto beans
>
> 2 oz. grated low-fat cheese
>
> Shredded lettuce
>
> Tomato
>
> 1 corn tortilla, cooked with nonstick spray

Burrito

> 1 whole wheat tortilla
>
> 1/2 cup black beans
>
> 1/2 cup fresh or canned salsa
>
> 2 oz. low-fat cheese

Chicken Breast and Vegetables

> 4 oz. skinless boneless chicken breast, baked with seasoning
>
> 1 cup green beans or other vegetable

WINNING DINNER OPTIONS

Chicken Dishes

Chicken Pesto, Vegetables and Brown Rice

6 oz. boneless chicken breast (raw weight)

1 Tbsp. pesto sauce

1 oz. low-fat cheese

Cut slits in the chicken and coat with pesto sauce. Place chicken and sauce under hot broiler, cook for 6 minutes (3 on each side). Top chicken with cheese and place under broiler until cheese melts.

1/2 cup brown rice or small baked potato

1 cup steamed vegetables

Broiled Chicken Breast, Lentils & Vegetables

5 oz. skinless boneless chicken breast

1/2 cup cooked lentils

1 cup fresh broccoli

1 cup fresh or frozen green beans

Spray the chicken with cooking spray and broil until tender. Serve with the cooked lentils and steamed or micro waved vegetables.

Lemon Chicken Breast

1 skinless boneless chicken thigh

Lemon juice

1/2 Tbsp. olive oil

1 shallot

1/2 Tbsp. capers

1 Tbsp. Dijon mustard

1 cup steamed vegetables

Combine lemon juice, olive oil, shallot, capers and Dijon mustard for a marinade. Place chicken in shallow roasting pan and cover with the sauce. Broil for 12–15 minutes until chicken is fully cooked.

Healthy Chicken Fingers & Vegetables

4 oz. chicken breast tenders

1 tsp. chili powder

1 tsp. ground cumin

1/4 tsp. salt

1 cup steamed vegetables

Combine chili powder, cumin, and salt; rub spice mixture onto chicken. Place chicken in a baking pan coated with cooking spray. Cook chicken in preheated oven at 350° F, 15 minutes, turning every 5 minutes. Serve with low-sugar BBQ sauce.

Healthy Fried Chicken

4 5-ounce chicken thighs, skinned

3/4 cup chicken broth

1 Tbsp. olive oil

1 cup toasted wheat germ

1 tsp. dried tarragon

1 tsp. dried rosemary, crushed

1 tsp. fresh parsley, chopped

1 tsp. garlic powder

Salt to taste

Preheat oven to 350° F. Pour chicken broth and olive oil in a small bowl. In another bowl, mix together the wheat germ, tarragon, rosemary, parsley, garlic powder, and salt. Dip the thighs, one at a time, in the broth-oil mixture, then coat with the wheat germ and herb mixture. Bake in oven until brown and cooked through, about 45–55 minutes.

Beef Dishes

Garlic Steak and Potato

6 oz. lean filet or sirloin steak

1 tsp. olive oil

3 cup cooked green beans

1/2 medium baked sweet potato or baked potato

For the Garlic Butter

1 oz. butter

1 clove crushed garlic

1 tsp. chopped fresh parsley

Black pepper

Brush the steak with the oil on sides, then grill or barbecue to taste. Put the butter in a small bowl and mix with the garlic, parsley, and pepper. Serve over cooked steak. Serve with cooked green beans and sweet potato.

1 cup steamed broccoli

Beef Tenderloin and Mashed Cauliflower

4 oz. grilled beef tenderloin

1 cup mixed salad greens

2 Tbsp. low-cal dressing

Mashed Cauliflower

1 medium head cauliflower, cut into florets

1 cup purified water

2 garlic cloves, minced

1 tsp. fresh chives, chopped

1/2 tsp. onion powder

1/2 tsp. fresh parsley, chopped

1 Tbsp. chicken or beef broth

In a medium pot, place cauliflower in water and bring to a quick boil. Lower heat to simmer and cover. Cook for an additional 12 minutes or until soft. Drain, transfer cauliflower to a bowl, and mash. Blend garlic, chives, onion powder, parsley, and broth with the mashed cauliflower. Serve hot.

London Broil with Mushrooms (4 servings)

1-1/2 lb. London broil, 1-inch thick

2 tsp. dried rosemary

4 cloves garlic, minced

2 Tbsp. extra virgin olive oil

1 cup sliced white mushrooms

Rub half the garlic and rosemary on each side of the meat. Heat olive oil in nonstick skillet over medium heat. Add steak; cook for 5 minutes on each side. Transfer meat to another plate. Add remaining ingredients; cook for about 4 minutes. Serve with salad.

1 cup mixed salad greens

2 Tbsp. low-cal dressing

Fish

Salmon Teriyaki & Vegetables

Teriyaki sauce (makes enough sauce for 2 servings)

1/4 cup reduced sodium tamari sauce

1/4 cup dry sherry

1 Tbsp. sesame oil

1 Tbsp. grated fresh ginger root

2 garlic cloves put through a garlic press

1 salmon fillet

Combine the ingredients for the marinade. Place the fish in a glass or ceramic dish, pour marinade over it, and marinate in the refrigerator for 2 hours. Preheat the broiler. Remove the fish from the marinade and transfer to a plate. Grill the fish, basting with the marinade, for 3–4 minutes. Turn and grill, basting again, for another 3–4 minutes. Do not overcook. Serve with salad or steamed vegetables. (Low-fat dressing 2 Tbsp.)

Ginger Salmon

4 oz. skinless salmon fillet

1/2 clove garlic

1/2 Tbsp. grated fresh ginger root

1 Tbsp. low-sodium soy sauce

1 green onion

Place salmon in shallow dish, pour marinade over fish. Bake at 350° F until fish flakes, 20–30 minutes, basting with pan juices. Serve with fresh steamed broccoli.

Trout

4 oz. whole trout

2 garlic cloves

Fresh or dried rosemary

1 lemon

Salt

Pepper

Season fish with salt and pepper; place rosemary, garlic, and lemon on fish. Broil for 5 minutes, turn, broil 5 minutes, until fish is cooked through. Serve with steamed vegetables.

Quick Fish Dish

4 oz. fish fillets

1 clove garlic, minced

Fresh mushroom caps

Chives

Parsley

2 Tbsp. Italian low-cal dressing

1 tsp. lemon juice

Cherry tomatoes or quartered tomatoes

Lightly oil shallow dish or spray with cooking spray. Place fish fillets in single layer. Mix dressing with garlic and lemon juice, pour over fish. Sprinkle with chives and parsley. Dip mushrooms and tomatoes in dressing and put in pan around fish. Bake at 350° F until fish flakes, 20–30 minutes, basting with pan juices. Serve with fresh steamed broccoli.

Tofu-Vegetable Stir-Fry

1 oz. extra-firm tofu, cubed

1 cup vegetables (bell peppers, mushrooms, onion, broccoli)

1/2 tsp. toasted sesame oil

Cooking spray

1 garlic clove

1/4 Tbsp. red pepper flakes

Spray wok or nonstick skillet with cooking spray. Add sesame oil and sauté red pepper flakes on medium-high heat; add garlic, onion, and vegetables. Cook for 2–3 minutes, add tofu and stir-fry until heated through.

Thai Tofu Stir-Fry

1 oz. extra-firm tofu, cubed

1/4 can light (no sugar added) coconut milk

1 clove garlic

1 cup vegetables (bok choy, celery, bell pepper, asparagus, mushrooms)

1/4 tsp. red pepper flakes

1 tsp. light soy sauce

1/2 Tbsp. lime juice

Fresh or dried basil to taste

Mix coconut milk, garlic, and lime juice in wok, heat on high. Add vegetables, cook for 10 minutes or until vegetables are cooked as desired. Add tofu and stir in soy sauce and basil.

SNACK TIME

Choose two snacks per day from list.

Snack Suggestion List:

1 serving fruit
1 serving string cheese
1 Tbsp. peanut butter with celery
1 Tbsp. peanut butter with one small apple
1 serving sugar-free Jell-O
1/2 oz. raw nuts
1 oz. roast turkey wrapped round celery or carrot sticks
3 oz. fresh tuna with 2 cups of lettuce
1/2 cup low-fat cottage cheese or yogurt
Cut-up veggies

Congratulations!

If you've stuck with the plan you should have reached your goal! You've done it! Celebrate your success! Take a few moments to think about the changes that have taken place with your body and health. Write down all of the things that have improved for you since you started the *Size 2 for Life* Program.

- Do you have more energy?

- How many pounds and inches have you lost?

- Are you stronger?

- Are you eating healthier?

- Has the way you look at your health changed?

- How have other areas of your life changed as your fitness changed?

Use this list as a reminder of your commitment to a healthy lifestyle. If you need extra motivation, keep a "before" photo as a reminder of all that you have accomplished.

Keeping the weight off permanently takes a daily commitment to leading a healthy lifestyle. Studies indicate that exercise is one of the most important things you can do for weight maintenance. To maintain your weight, use the tools that worked for you as you lost the weight: eating healthy meals and snacks, eating low-calorie, nutrient-dense foods, weighing yourself weekly to detect small weight gains before they become larger, using a journal to help you recognize any setbacks and to stay in control of your eating and exercise habits.

Continue to move forward and focus on all the wonderful benefits of your healthy lifestyle. Continue to share your success stories with us and inspire others to join the program.

Stay in touch at: www.size2forlife.com

Appendices – Easy copy forms

1. Preparing for the 21-Day Size 2 for Life Diet & Fitness Program – Strategic Plan

2. Personal Success Contract

3. Train Like An Athlete Action Foods

4. Sample Shopping List

5. Fitness Check Sheet – Evening Program

Preparing for the 21-Day *Size 2 for Life* Diet & Fitness Program

Strategic Plan

"People with goals succeed because they know where they are going." - Earl Nightingale

The first step in making a real commitment is your belief in yourself; "I am doing this," instead of "I'm going to try to do it." The language you use is just as important as your physical actions. Create an inner and outer dialogue that is focused on the results you want. Know that you have the power to change your behavior and create the outcome you desire.

Take a few minutes to answer the following questions writing down the first three answers that come to mind:

Why do you want to change your body?

 1.

 2.

 3.

What is preventing you from achieving your goal?

 1.

 2.

 3.

Personal Success Contract

I, _____, commit to starting my fitness program today, _____.

I commit to using the Size 2 for Life – Change Your Life Workout Program consistently and following the Size 2 for Life healthful eating program that will help me attain my fitness and health goals.

I will only fuel my body with the most nutritious foods possible.

I will be kind to myself and appreciate all that my body does for me.

I will strive to challenge my body and my mind.

I will acknowledge and reward myself for my achievements along the way.

_____

Signature

Sample Shopping List

Fresh Vegetables

_____

Lettuce
Other Greens
Cucumbers
Carrots
Asparagus
Zucchini
Radishes
Tomatoes
Green Beans
Onions
Green Onions
Peppers
Cauliflower
Broccoli
Peas
Celery
Potatoes
Corn
Sweet Potatoes
Squash
Other Vegetables:

_____

_____

_____

Fresh Fruits

Bananas
Apples
Oranges
Pears
Peaches
Nectarines
Grapefruit
Berries
Other Fruits:

_____

_____

Frozen Foods

Green Beans
Mixed Vegetables
Chicken Breasts
Fruit Juice Bars
Blueberries
Corn
Fish Fillets
Onions
Vegetarian Burgers
Other Frozen Foods

_____

_____

_____

Canned Foods

Black Beans
Tomatoes
Marinara Sauce
Tuna
Salmon
Pinto Beans
White Beans
Pineapple
Other Canned Foods:

_____

_____

_____

Meats

Lean Hamburger
Steaks
Fish
Shellfish
Chicken
Turkey

Ham
Other Meats:

_____

_____

_____

Grains and Cereals

Whole Grain Bread
Whole Grain Cereal
Oatmeal
Whole Wheat or Fat-Free Tortillas
High-fiber Cereal (Kashi)
Other Grains:

_____

_____

_____

Beverages

Water
Coffee
Herb Tea
Green Tea
Other Beverages:

_____

_____

Dairy and Eggs

Low-Fat/Nonfat Sour Cream
Low-Fat/Nonfat Milk
Egg Whites
String Cheese
Low-Fat Cream Cheese
L/N Yogurt
FAGE Nonfat Greek Yogurt

Other Dairy:

_____

Soy/Vegetarian Options

Tofu
Light or low-fat Soy Milk
Tempeh
Vegetarian Burger Patties (i.e. Boca Burgers)

_____

_____

Miscellaneous Items

Protein Powder, Whey, Hemp or Soy
Psyllium
Bragg Liquid Aminos
WASA Crackers
Stevia
Flaxseed Meal and/or Flaxseed Oil
Low-Fat Dressings
Mustard
Almonds
Peanut Butter
Pecans
Olive Oil Cooking Spray
Garlic
Popcorn
Salsa
Other Miscellaneous Items:

_____

_____

_____

Ashley's Favorite Fitness Finds!

Daily Plate is an awesome FREE website that tracks your daily calories.
http://www.thedailyplate.com/

Eat Right provides information on nutrition. Eatright.org

National Institute of Health http://www.nih.gov/ This is a great site if to get information on health issues and new scientific research.

Exercise TV http://exercisetv.tv/ ExerciseTV is a free website offering hundreds of fat burning workouts like cardio, abs, yoga, dance and more!

iTunes Podrunner Free workout music mixes.
http://itunes.apple.com/WebObjects/MZStore.woa/wa/viewPodcast?id=272591768

lululemon athletic http://www.lululemon.com High quality fitness apparel company. They also offer free instore classes and community events.

Fitness Check Sheet – Evening Program

Aerobics

Arrive at the gym and begin with a five-minute warm up on either a bicycle or elliptical, if available.

Move over to a treadmill and make sure you again stretch out those gastrocs, etc.

Begin the Step-It-Up component as in the morning exercise, and increase you pace in increments until you're jogging at 4.0–4.5 miles per hour (or greater, depending on your progress) for five-minute segments again.

Begin the Step-It-Down sequence and decrease your pace at the same rate as the morning program.

Stretch out a bit. Congratulations! The aerobic component of your workout is done.

Toning

Exercise	Reps	Weight	Exercise	Reps	Weight
Crunches			Rotational weighted abdominals		
Overhead press machine			Angled forward press		
Biceps curls			Upper back pulls (row)		
Deltoid lifts			Lumbar (lower) back extensions		
Crunch machine			Gastrocnemius (lower leg) lifts		
Pectoral flies			Gluteus (leg) presses		
Forward press			Quadriceps (leg) extensions		
Full extension fly machine (if available)			Hamstring (leg) curls		
Backward fly's			Leg abductions		
Overhead pull			Leg adductions		
Free weight curls					

References and Resources

Consumer Reports, "Dangerous Supplements Still at Large," 5/2004. Consumers Union Publications.

Consumer Reports, "Comparisons of Diets," 2006.

The Musculoskeletal Manual, Bernbaum.

American Journal of Clinical Nutrition: "Physical activity and weight loss: does prescribing higher physical activity improve outcome?" October 2003. Jeffery, Wing, Sherwood and Tate.

Medicine & Science in Sports & Exercise: "Influence of exercise training on physiological and performance changes with weight loss in men." Kraemer, et al.

"Psycho-Cyb The Spread of Obesity in a Large Social Network over 32 Years." Nicholas A. Christakis, M.D., Ph.D., M.P.H., and James H. Fowler, Ph.D. ernetics, Dr Maxwell Maltz. *The New England Journal of Medicine*, July 26, 2007.

Williams MA, Haskell WL, Ades PA, et al. "Resistance exercise in individuals with and without cardiovascular disease": 2007. *Circulation* 2007; DOI: 10.1161/CIRCULATION AHA.107.185214. Available at: www.circulationaha.org.

US Department of Health and Human Services. "Physical Activity and Health: A Report of the Surgeon General." Atlanta, Georgia: US Department of Health and Human Services, Centers for Disease Control and Prevention, National Center for Chronic Disease Prevention and Health Promotion; 1996.

"American College of Sports Medicine Position Stand: the recommended quantity and quality of exercise for developing and maintaining cardiorespiratory and muscular fitness and flexibility in healthy adults." *Med Sci Sports Exerc*. 1998; 30: 975–991.

"Leisure Activities and the Risk of Dementia in the Elderly." *New England Journal of Medicine*. Joe Verghese, M.D., Richard B. Lipton, M.D., Mindy J. Katz, M.P.H., Charles B. Hall, Ph.D., Carol A. Derby, Ph.D., Gail Kuslansky, Ph.D., Anne F. Ambrose, M.D., Martin Sliwinski, Ph.D., and Herman Buschke, M.D.

"How to Keep Your Aging Brain Fit: Aerobics," *The Wall Street Journal*, by Sharon Begley, November 16, 2006.

William D. McArdle, Frank J. Katch, Victor L. Katch, *Exercise Physiology, Energy, Nutrition & Human Performance*, Sixth Edition, 2007 Chapter 28: "Body Composition Assessment."

The Authors

Ashley Marriott has been designing and instructing dance and fitness programs for more than 10 years and is the creator of *Burn 'N Firm*, a popular DVD fitness dance workout series. She is dedicated to using her experience and energy to educate and encourage women and has helped thousands of people to reach their weight loss and fitness goals. Her classes and trainings reach a broad range of clients that include working moms, celebrities, active seniors and professionals who all share the desire to get fit, have fun, and lead healthier lives.

Ashley is a frequent guest on radio and television sharing her get fit strategies and she has written dozens of fitness and nutrition articles for publications worldwide. She continues to teach packed classes throughout Los Angeles bringing an infectious enthusiasm to all of her classes and training sessions.

Ashley holds certifications in Personal Training, Group Fitness, Nutrition and is certified by the *National Academy of Sports Medicine*, Aerobics *and Fitness Association of America and is a member of I.D.E.A.*

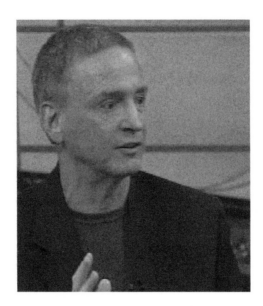

Marc L. Paulsen, M.D. is a graduate of Brandeis University and Stanford University Medical School. He received his training at University of California, Irvine Medical Center as well as course work in Epidemiology through The Division of Public Health at the Medical College of Wisconsin. His practice has included Emergency Medicine, Occupational Medicine and General Family Medicine. He is a member of the American Academy of Sports Medicine and a former Medical Director of the Exercise Science Lab at Orange Coast College in California. He has been featured as an expert guest on numerous radio and TV shows in the United States and Canada including ABC, CBS, NBC, FOX, CNN and KTLA/CW.

Index